P9-CJX-941

The Wonder of It All

THE WONDER OF IT ALL

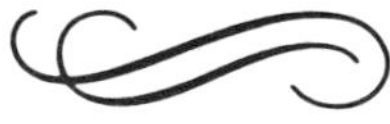

Jeanne Logue

HARPER & ROW, PUBLISHERS

New York, Hagerstown, San Francisco,

London, Sydney

THE WONDER OF IT ALL. Copyright © 1979 by Jeanne Logue. All rights reserved. Printed in the United States of America. No part of this book may be used or reproduced in any manner whatsoever without written permission except in the case of brief quotations embodied in critical articles and reviews. For information address Harper & Row, Publishers, Inc., 10 East 53rd Street, New York, N.Y. 10022. Published simultaneously in Canada by Fitzhenry & Whiteside Limited, Toronto, and simultaneously in Australia–New Zealand by Harper & Row (Australasia) Pty. Ltd., and simultaneously in the United Kingdom by Harper & Row Ltd., London.

FIRST EDITION

Designed by C. Linda Dingler

Drawings by Lynda West

Library of Congress Cataloging in Publication Data

Logue, Jeanne.
The wonder of it all.

1. Logue, Jeanne. 2. Veterinarians—New York (State)—Biography. 3. Veterinary medicine—New York (State) I. Title.
SF613.L6A33 636.089′092′4 [B] 78–20175
ISBN (U.S.A. and Canada) 0–06–012654–X
ISBN (except U.S.A. and Canada) 0–06–337005–0

79 80 81 82 83 10 9 8 7 6 5 4 3 2 1

This book is lovingly dedicated to my mother, Carrie Pfister Neubecker, without whose quiet strength and patient understanding so many things would not have been possible.

Acknowledgments

My knowledge and understanding of veterinary medicine has been acquired through the work of many people who lived before my time, people who devoted their whole lifetime to the study of the causation, transmission and treatment of those diseases affecting not only animals but also those diseases which are transmitted from animals to man.

My debt of gratitude goes back almost four thousand years to Salihotra, the first recorded veterinarian in history, who practiced in India around 1800 B.C. during the Vedic Age. A rich heritage lies in his knowledge and skill in the use of over 700 medicinal plants and more than 100 surgical instruments. Salihotra, who wrote in Sanskrit, accurately recorded his work in what now must be the most ancient of all veterinary journals. His animal health programs were not left to religious ritual and superstition. While he revered animal life and believed in the reincarnation of all living creatures, he never confused his religion with science.

Around the turn of this century the work of Dr. Cooper Curtice championed the theory that the southern cattle tick, Margaropus annulatus, was the sole carrier of the disease known as Texas Fever. This veterinarian made an epochal breakthrough in medical history when he eventually proved that arthropods were capable of acting as carriers of mammalian diseases. It is to a mentality and a sense of dedication such as this that I owe a further debt of gratitude.

More contemporarily still, I acknowledge with deep appreciation the sound education I received from all my professors at the New York State College of Veterinary Medicine at Cornell University. I cannot name them all, but I especially remember the enthusiasm of Dr. Hagan, then the dean of the veterinary college and the head of the bacteriology department, the vivaciousness of dynamic Dr. Danks, head of large animal medicine and surgery, the humor or Dr. Stephensen, head of the small animal division, the austerity of Dr. Olafsen, chief pathologist, the dedication of Dr. Miller, head of anatomy, the gentleness of Dr. Hayden, head of physical chemistry, the meticulousness of Dr. Dukes, head of physiology, and last but not least, the joie de vivre of all my classmates!

I thank my sister Marjorie Neubecker who helped me type this manuscript for as long as she was able, and my daughter-in-law Antoinette Logue, who carried on with this task after Marjorie died.

I will never forget the kindness shown to me by my friend Dr. Ruth Nanda Anshen, philosopher, author and editor. I acknowledge that, but for Dr. Anshen, this manuscript may never have been called to the attention of Buz Wyeth and Steve Roos, editors at Harper & Row. I wish to thank all the people at Harper & Row who have had anything to do with helping me in this exciting venture—the publication of my first book.

The most immediate moment of appreciation, an appreciation that I am aware of every day of my life, goes to my family. It is my hope that the great love and respect I have for them somehow shines through in this book.

A glossary of medical terms will be found on page 204.

The Wonder of It All

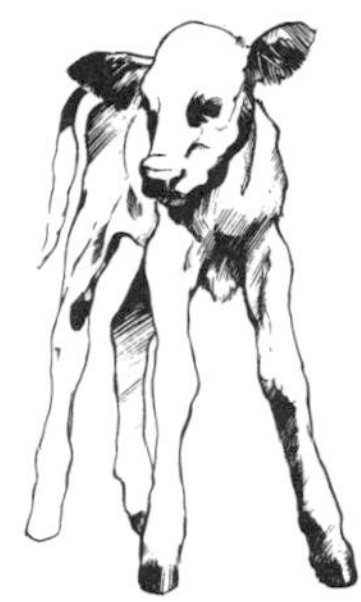

1

In my dream I stood alone in the center of the field. A warm breeze tugged at my hair as it did at the wild flowers, making their velvet anthers quiver on their slender filaments. Crisscrossing this field of flowers was a network of paths which converged randomly, and then diverged again into various wayward directions. Gradually over the horizon all manner of animals came, each taking its own path toward me. Sometimes the paths were so close that the animals touched each other along their way. They were always aware of one another, but this did not seem to distract them as they plodded steadily toward the center of the field. Brushing by me in their passage, they continued on their way, eventually to disappear over the opposite horizon. I felt a strange oneness with them all. Next, from the distance, I heard the soft dong of a cowbell and I watched a huge white cow as she approached me. As she lumbered nearer, the sound of her bell grew louder and the interval between clangs grew shorter and shorter, until, as she came quite close, each clang blurred itself into the next one and the sound changed into a steady ringing. The sound became annoying now, louder and very persistent, until suddenly, with a start, I awakened and reached for the bedside phone.

Fully awake now, I picked up the receiver and said, "Dr. Logue speaking."

"This is John Hansen, Doctor. I'm sorry to wake you, but you remember that cow I had such trouble breeding? Well, she's been in labor since nine-fifteen last night. I thought maybe everything would be all right, but something has gone wrong. She's stopped straining—hasn't done a thing for the past four hours. Could you please come?"

The glowing hands of the clock pointed accusingly in the dark to 4:30 A.M.

"Sure, John, I'll be there. What's this now—her third calf?"

"Yes."

"She's never had any trouble calving before, has she?"

"Nope. Everything went without a hitch."

"Right. I'll get dressed and be there as soon as I can."

"We'll have all the lights on for you. Thanks a lot, Doctor."

I placed the receiver in its cradle and rolled over for one last warm snuggle against my husband, while I tried to prod him into consciousness enough for me to tell him that I was on my way.

"Joe! Joe, wake up! I've got to go. Are you awake enough to hear me? If I'm not back by the time the alarm goes off, get up and wake Raymond for school. Honey, do you hear me?"

"Mm . . . yes, I'm awake." And then, "Jesus H. Christ! What time is it?"

"Four-thirty." I was out of bed now, already in my underwear and stepping into heavy work pants.

"Can't it wait until morning?"

"'Fraid not." My answer was muffled as I pulled a sweater over my head. "It's John Hansen—a case of dystocia. We might lose that calf if we wait. Don't forget to wake Ray. His school clothes are all laid out and ready. Bye-bye, now. I love you." I leaned over and kissed him.

But there was no response. Joe had already fallen back into a sound sleep.

I always kept the trunk of the car packed for wee-hour emergencies such as this. It not only saved time when I was in a rush, but also there was less chance of my forgetting something if supplies were put in place during a moment of unhurried deliberation. The only two things I had to pick up on my way out were the box from the office refrigerator containing vials of antibiotics, hormones and vaccines, and a carton from the shelf above containing flasks of calcium gluconate, saline and Ringer's lactate—an assortment of various solutions of electrolytes for intravenous administration. I always took two or more of each type of solution when I went on farm calls because the glass flasks, cool from being in a cold car, would "sweat" when they were in a warm barn for a while and they would become slippery. Being large and awkward to hold, they could easily slip from my grasp and break while I was preparing them for use. It was much better, I had decided long ago, to reach for that handy second flask if I broke the first one, rather than drive all the way back to the office for a replacement.

I was on my way now, driving in the darkness, thinking of the calf I was going to have to pull. It seemed like only yesterday that John was trying to breed this animal. It didn't seem possible that about 290 days had gone by. I mused on the variances in the gestation periods of the different breeds of cows, which range from 281 to 290 days. I used to think a cow was a cow and they'd all be the same.

I thought about the Brown Swiss breed and was glad to have John Hansen as my client. He had a fine herd and his animals and barns were well cared for and always clean. Besides, the Brown Swiss was my favorite breed, beautiful with their cinnamon-light to darker-brown bodies, their creamy briskets and jet-black noses and black tail brushes. And their soulful eyes! No animal face on earth, I felt, so completely exemplified the eternal feminine as the face of a Brown Swiss cow.

Lights, seen through the cold air, twinkled in the distance; they grew brighter and twinkled less as I drew closer to the farm. I turned into the driveway and drove up the lane, which was bordered on either side by well-matched mature Scotch pines, obviously planted with thoughtful care many years ago. John was waiting for me by the barn. I got out of the car and opened the trunk.

"Hi, John. Anything interesting happening?"

"No. Everything's the same. Here, let me carry that heavy bag."

I thanked him as I balanced the carton containing the flasks on my left hip and secured a second instrument bag in my right hand. Entering the barn, I remember, I said something very profound, like, "Well, let's see what's what."

"Can you give her a shot to make her start laboring again?" John asked as he carefully placed the bag he was carrying on the floor outside a roomy stall which he used as his "delivery room."

"I could," I answered as I placed my gear next to the bag John had been carrying, "but since she was in forceful labor before and couldn't expel the calf, something must be wrong. Before I go injecting anything, I'd better take a look to find why she's having trouble this time."

Quickly I poured disinfectant into a bucket, and after diluting it with water, I washed the cow's rear, cleansing it of small flecks of fecal material and any urine or mucus that had dried on the vaginal tuft of hair. Next, I put my left arm into a long rubber obstetrical glove which came up to my shoulder, and I stretched the shoulder strap over my head and under my right armpit to anchor it. Lifting aside the animal's tail, I gently slipped my gloved hand between the lips of the vulva, into the warm vagina, through the firm cervix and into the body of the uterus, where I made contact with two tiny hoofs, which were almost cartilaginous and yielded to my touch. I moved my hand along the calf's forelegs, slid past the shoulder and along the neck, where I could feel the pulsating carotid artery.

"It's still alive, John! I can feel its pulse!" and I kept exploring until I found the cause of the trouble—the grotesque angle of the calf's head. It was twisted upward and back, with the jawbone and chin tilted and caught fast, jammed against the mother's bony pelvis. All during the long hours of the beast's labor, each successive muscular heave had only served to wedge the little calf's head more tightly against the bony pelvic prison.

By now the great cow was very tired; her muscles were fatigued, almost flaccid and yielding, and this enabled me to back the calf away from the pelvis. I managed to push it forward into the mother's body, free its head, straighten its neck and position it for delivery.

"Now's the time for that injection, John," and I explained what had happened. "If I'd given the injection before straightening the calf, it would only have made matters worse. Now that the calf is in proper alignment, we can proceed with the business at hand." I injected a dose of posterior pituitary extract deep into the muscle of the cow's rump to stimulate uterine contraction. Now I gloved my right arm, washed with disinfectant and turned to tend the animal. I inserted my left hand again and rested it on the calf's head, to guide it through the birth canal when the cow started contractions.

The barn was very quiet now. No more splashing of water, rattling of buckets or even the clink of a bottle or vial as the three of us patiently waited. The cow was a statue of stillness, with only her swollen belly moving slowly in and out, as though the beast knew to conserve her energy and not waste it on useless movements.

Five minutes passed, six, and then there was a faint but distinct tightening of pressure on my hand inside the cow.

Straw rustled softly as the animal changed her position slightly and braced her hind legs. She breathed a sigh and a soft lowing sound flowed with it, but then all placidity was gone, for the beast was alive now to her task as she sucked in a huge tidal volume of air to sustain her during her first contraction. The smooth muscle fibers of the uterus started a wave of contraction, and with wondrous synchronization the striated abdominal and intercostal muscles contracted too, and their concerted straining forced the calf closer to the exit of the birth canal. The contraction spent itself and there was another huge intake of air, which sucked the calf away from the opening again, as an ocean wave receding from the shore sucks a floating log which it had almost deposited safely on the sand back into the sea. There was another contraction. The calf rode the wave; its feet surged into the pelvis and the little head forcefully, yet gently, bumped against my waiting hand, for the calf was still cushioned by several gallons of placental fluid, the membranes having not yet broken. Again there was the receding tide, another gulp of air and another powerful push. The calf was more insistent now, demanding to be born, and with the next cushioned bump my hand slipped behind the calf's head and I was able to tuck it down and forward between the front legs to prepare the new creature for its dive into this world.

There being no further fear of the head being caught at an odd angle, I quickly used both my hands and grasped the calf behind its elbows, holding fast. The laboring cow's next gasp for air caused a strong negative pressure within her abdominal cavity, but I kept a firm hold and this time my prize was not sucked back into the caverns of the deep. It was a tight fit for the calf, its fluids, the mother's pelvic bone and me. It felt as though there were a tourniquet on both my forearms and my hands began to swell. And so, inexorably, the unrelenting struggle continued, with alternating gasping intakes of air and forceful bearings down.

By this time the farmer and I, without realizing it, were suspending our breathing and then grunting in empathy with the cow whenever she held her breath or strained and pushed in her powerful efforts to expel her calf. John happened to catch my eye, and suddenly we were both laughing.

"Isn't it funny?" John said. "Every time I catch myself straining along with the animal, and every time I realize how silly and useless it is and I swear I will never do it again, but every time I catch myself doing it again!"

"Me, too!" I laughed and tossed my head slightly in an effort to shift my position. The stiff hair on the cow's rump was beginning to itch my face as I clung to that calf, literally cheek to cheek with its mother.

"I'm sure I can pull this calf all by myself, John. I doubt if we'll need any ropes. One or two more good heaves will do it." I assumed my usual pretzel-like position in preparation for the most difficult part of the delivery, that of getting the head and shoulders through the pelvic canal. Planting my left foot firmly on the floor and balancing on that leg, I brought my right leg up so that my knee was next to my ear, and I placed my right foot squarely against the cow's behind, just to the right of her tail. The next time the cow strained, I pulled on the calf and at the same time pushed myself slowly away from the cow with all my might. I maintained this tension until the cow's next contraction, at which time I pushed myself still farther from the cow, pulling her calf with me.

The cow's knees buckled under her heavy body and suddenly there was a flood as her membranes ruptured, and on this welling tide, with a splash, the calf's front legs, then its head, were out. The lips of the cow's vulva, stretched almost paper thin now, looked like a bandanna tied around the calf's head.

With another heave and a pull, the shoulders followed and the calf was out up to its chest.

"There, now. Isn't that a relief, Serena?" I asked the cow, and she responded to her name with a soft low. It was the first sound she had made during this entire procedure.

"So rest yourself a moment, Sociable Serena," I suggested to her, calling her by her full name. But really, I had no need to say this, for the beast already knew exactly what to do. Serena sighed and rested and patiently waited, preparing herself for the next onslaught of contractions.

Soon enough it began again. I cradled the calf's head and shoulders in my arms and John stepped up and caught the hips and rear legs of the calf as it slithered out in a gush of placental fluid and foam—an exquisitely perfect little creature, I thought, born from foam like a bovine Aphrodite.

The umbilical cord of a calf is very short compared to that of a foal or a human, and because of its shortness, it invariably ruptures within the vagina of the cow during birth due to one of the more vigorous movements of either the mother or the calf. Serena turned about now, alive to the needs of her calf. She started nuzzling it and licking its moist navel with her powerful, rasplike tongue. The urachus, through which the calf had urinated before it was born, as well as the left and right umbilical arteries, were already within the calf's abdominal cavity, about an inch or two from the umbilical ring. There was no fear of bleeding, for the retraction of the stumps of the arteries served to thicken the walls of the vessels sufficiently to close their lumens, and the rupture by linear tension had frayed the broken ends. This, along with the inverted tough connective tissue drawn from the umbilical ring, effectively barred any hemorrhage from the broken arteries. The umbilical vein, on the other hand, had ruptured just *outside* the umbilical ring, and having a very thin, inelastic wall, did not markedly retract at all but remained dangling outside the body wall like a tattered little rag. The umbilical vein is not supplied with valves, as are most veins, so all the residual blood trapped within the stump of the calf's vessel spontaneously drained away.

Marveling at nature's way, I watched that cow with love and reverence as she continued to clean the birth wound, removing all the viscous Whartonian jelly and bits of blood. This dried the wound and rendered it less susceptible to infection. Serena gently butted her newborn calf, causing it to move and to breathe more deeply. She licked and slurped all the mucus from the calf's nose and lips, then returned to licking the navel, removing the last jewel of jelly, then up along the ribs again, massaging the calf, continuing her Turkish-towel rub with her tongue until the new creature was glowing and dry and gleaming in the light that was shining from the ceiling above the stall. The calf's little hoofs no longer appeared to be cartilaginous now; they were hard and shiny, black like coal, reminding me of four new black patent leather spats.

Naturally, I had to try to improve on nature, and when fastidious Serena stopped fussing at her calf, I asked John to support the calf in a standing position. Holding a jar of tincture of iodine in my hand, I placed the wide mouth of the jar against the abdominal floor so as to submerge the navel stump in the liquid. The two of us stood over the calf, while I continued this submersion for a good three minutes. I said, "It's a nice heifer calf, John. She'll probably produce as much milk as her mother someday."

"She'll have to produce some to keep up with Sociable Serena," John replied, with a laugh that erased all remaining lines of tension from his face. "Serena produced over thirteen hundred pounds of milk and six hundred pounds of butter fat last year. She's my prize cow."

We next held the new calf on its back and I dusted the navel liberally with a mixture of powdered alum and iodoform.

"How's your supply of iodoform holding out?" I asked.

"I think you'd better let me have a few more containers. I'm using my last one now and it's over half empty."

"Remember to dust the stump of the cord frequently until the cord is thoroughly dry. You know the stump's a great avenue of infection."

"I know. And I'll muzzle the young calves when I place them together so they don't suck on each other." John was referring to the tendency of calves, especially young dairy calves, to seize upon each other's protruding parts—scrotum, teats or navel stumps—just after feeding and suck vigorously.

"I'm going to tell Inga the good news. We'll bring coffee. I know she has the pot on." And John hurried to the farmhouse. There was no doubt about his Nordic parentage, with his fair but weathered complexion and wintery blue eyes. He was tall and heavy-boned, yet lean, a man of about forty-five whose blond hair had not darkened much with age. He had about him a self-assured, well-coordinated grace and had a lithe walk in spite of a decided limp, the result of a serious wound, received in 1918 during the First World War, which had almost resulted in the loss of his right leg. I was most intrigued by the man's hands. They were enormous. They seemed to be all knuckles. They were calloused and the cuticles grew down somewhat upon nails that were short from being broken, not cut or filed. But the nails were always clean; I can't remember ever seeing them dirty. In spite of their bigness, John's fingers were extremely dexterous, and his hands could be as gentle as a woman's if the occasion arose.

I had just about collected all my gear and was about to wash my boots in the barnyard with disinfectant and change into other shoes when John and his wife, Inga, appeared. John was holding a big blue metal percolator with a heavy red potholder and Inga was holding three coffee mugs hooked through the handles with the fingers of one hand, her other hand carrying a plate covered with a napkin.

"Here, now, Jeanne. I'll clean those boots for you. You go on into the barn with Inga and gather the rest of your stuff together and enjoy your coffee," John ordered.

"Well, O.K. Thanks!" He didn't have to twist my arm on that one, and I slipped out of my big clumsy boots and put on a pair of sneakers.

"Have you ever noticed," Inga asked, "how John always uses 'Doc' when he calls you on business or during a work period, but lapses into 'Jeanne' when the doctoring is over?"

"Yes, like now, when we have coffee, or if we're at someone's home for the evening. I wonder if he realizes that he switches names. I like it. I like being called by my first name." And I took another delicious bite of muffin. Inga's muffins were made with bran, pumpkin and dates, and I had tried unsuccessfully to duplicate her recipe. I supposed mine never tasted as good because Inga cooked and strained fresh pumpkins from the farm, while I used the canned stuff bought in the store.

I noticed that she looked tired and worn and told her so, and I asked if something was wrong.

"I'm fine, really, Jeanne. I guess I'm just letting John Junior's bad arm upset me. That boy's constantly on my mind, the last one I think of before I go to sleep and my first thought as soon as I wake up."

Inga's only son, Johnnie, had been seriously injured on Iwo Jima during World War II. Attempting to burrow into the volcanic sand on the beach to escape the hail of enemy fire from gun positions on Mount Suribachi, Johnnie had had practically his entire shoulder ripped off, and the Hansens were now coming to the chilling realization that their son would probably never have any useful degree of movement in his arm.

"It's like reliving a nightmare." Inga sighed with a tired wave of her hand. "The first war my husband, the second war my son. That battle of Iwo Jima lasted from February nineteenth all the way to March sixteenth. I thought it would never end. The whole war was over by September second, but that was five months too late for Johnnie. He's still not well and I worry so about his recurrent fevers and his bouts of infection."

I sympathized with Inga and could understand her grieving. I don't think there is anything more wearing or spirit-sapping than having one thing constantly on your mind and not being able to do much of anything about it.

John had returned to the barn in time to hear Inga's remarks. She handed him a cup of coffee. He peered into the steaming cup a moment and then said, "I wish this time it really could have been the war to end all wars and you wouldn't have to face the prospect of going through one with your children, Jeanne." He took a gulp of coffee and continued: "I hate to say it, but I'd be naïve if I let myself really believe there will be lasting peace. Give us another twenty-five to fifty years—"

"Speaking of children," I interrupted, for suddenly I could not wait to get back home. "I must go. Right now! I always try to get back home before Raymond leaves for school or Joe goes off to work. Otherwise, what with afternoon office hours, I won't see anyone, except little Marilyn, until almost dinnertime—and even that's usually interrupted with one thing or another." I put down my coffee mug and thanked Inga.

When the car was packed and I was turning out of the driveway, I called to John.

"Be sure to let me know if the cow hasn't cleaned within six hours. Anything after six hours with a cow can be considered as a retained placenta."

"I'll watch her, Doc. And thanks again for coming so fast and at such a miserable hour."

"You're welcome, John. Y' know? If I had a nice calf like that, I'd name her Pasiphaë."

And I was on my way, driving fast, in hopes of having some time to spend with my family before they were all scattered by the winds of the day's activities. The sun was just beginning to rise, a little farther to the north than the day before, since spring was on its way in Kingston, New York. Buds on bushes and trees were not swollen yet, but a little close inspection revealed that they were not quite so shrunken and shriveled with cold as they had been. Rhododendron and laurel leaves, which had been tightly curled, shivering all winter, were beginning to relax a bit, and like so many anxiously furrowed brows showing relief from harassment, were becoming smooth and serene again, expanding in warm and secure thoughts of springtime.

Joe and I never have had spring fever; quite the other way. Springtime has always charged us both with a fresh flow of energy and an urgent desire to finish old jobs, tackle new and try even harder to do everything more perfectly.

Suddenly, as I pulled into our driveway that morning, I experienced such a euphoric mood that I had to pause a moment before getting out of the car. What caused this delicious sense of well-being, anyway? I tried hard to locate the origin of this mood so that perhaps I might recreate it sometime in the future as a booster if I ever felt low or melancholy and needed a renewal of the spirits.

But as I tried to analyze my state of mind the euphoria faded away, for I had tried to pick apart a frail, intangible thing and in its dissection had lost it. I sighed, convinced that any future dividends of this moment could be gained only by making a withdrawal from my memory bank. I did make two mental bank deposits that morning. The first was a very tangible welling up of love every time I thought of my family; the second was my love and sustained enthusiasm for my profession. Both were deposits of purest gold.

I quickly replaced the various vials in the refrigerator,

slammed the door shut, ran through the waiting room and into the vestibule, which served office and house. I picked up Raymond's boots, worn the day before, and tossed them into the closet as I passed by, and at last went through the door into the kitchen. I could hear family activity upstairs, so I went to the foot of the stairs and yelled, "Guess what?"

Raymond immediately appeared, leaning over the banister, with toothbrush clamped between his molar teeth.

"You're back! That's what!" and he inhaled and tilted his head back quickly as white toothpaste froth almost spilled over his lower lip.

"Don't talk with your mouth full of toothpaste, Raymond," his father directed as he came out of the bedroom clad only in a pair of shorts.

"You could get inhalation pneumonia that way, but what's worse, you'll stain our carpet if any spills. Go spit it out and finish dressing. Hi, Jeanne. How did things go?" Joe directed this last to me while drying himself roughly behind his neck and ears. When Joe washed, it was never a light rinse, a little cat-wash type of thing; rather, it was like a surgical scrub in its harshness and thoroughness.

Joe is an electrical engineer and I can't think of anything he ever does that is done in a superficial way. His is a complex personality; he is a meticulous and fastidious man who demands high standards from himself and from others. He possesses a keen intelligence and has a rare combination of abilities, being as sharp in his abstract thinking and reasoning as he is skilled in his dexterity and his mechanical sense. As I stood at the bottom of the staircase that morning, I absolutely adored him. I was convinced my husband was a genius, was sure his corporation, IBM, didn't nearly appreciate all his many talents, and that there wasn't anything under the sun that he could not do perfectly if he put his mind to it.

Joe is slightly under six feet tall, has black curly hair and penetrating dark-brown eyes. His eyes are very active and dart as he talks as if trying to keep up with his racing thoughts. Sometimes, when Joe smiles, his eyes seem to change color, turning a lighter shade of brown; warmth will suddenly shine through, then disappear just as suddenly when his smile is gone. He is a well-developed, muscular man, like a powerful sycamore tree, and he is good when it comes to athletics—a fact that for some reason surprises colleagues who don't know him well.

I noted the strong movements of my husband's large deltoid muscles as he dried himself, and in answer to his question I told him, "Fine, Joe. The calf's head was jammed. I'll see about breakfast. I'm sure I heard Mame come in just now. Will you be down soon?"

"In about ten minutes. Raymond too. Marilyn's in bed, playing with a doll."

I returned to the kitchen and said good morning to Mame, our housekeeper, who was fighting with a doorknob on the hall closet door in an effort to open the door and hang up her coat.

Mame finally joined me in the kitchen, and tying an apron around her waist, she remarked, "Looks like you've been out already, Dr. Logue, from what I see of those white pants you have on. I'll wash them for you when I get breakfast out of the way."

"Thank you, Mame. I've been on the go since four-thirty this morning. Just got back home. I'll put the coffee pot on, and you start the rest of the breakfast. I'll change into clean clothes and get Marilyn dressed."

"Seems to me that's all you do," stated Mame dryly, "change from large-animal clothes into small-animal clothes. Can't you arrange it so you do all your farm calls at one time and then do just small-animal work here at the hospital for the rest of the day?"

"It certainly would be a more efficient way to parcel time, but if a call comes at one o'clock in the afternoon from some farmer, I can't very well say, 'Sorry, I've done my large-animal stint for the day—can't come.' Suppose it was a case of milk fever? That would need immediate attention—it couldn't possibly wait until the next day."

"Well, I think it's terrible! People coming and going all the time. You were in that office till late last night. Now you've been up since four-thirty and will be going full tilt till late tonight again. People don't show no consideration. I don't see how you can keep it up." Mame sounded abused.

"It's not so bad, Mame. Remember that it's almost springtime, when my batteries get recharged! In the spring, I never get tired."

I chatted with Marilyn as I helped her get dressed.

"I'll button the three buttons down the back of your jumper, then you can get into your slacks while I change my clothes. O.K., Marilyn?"

"I don't know how," Marilyn quickly replied.

"Why, Marilyn, of course you do! You've gotten into your slacks before, all by yourself."

"But I forget, Mommy." I knew that Marilyn hadn't really forgotten, for her chin was on her chest, her eyes were averted and her voice was almost a whisper. Then her head shot up, and with a smile of sweet accord, as though a bright new idea had just presented itself, she suggested, "Why don't you show me *again,* Mommy? You know," she said persuasively, "how you laid them on the floor for me with the label up so I could sit on the floor and stick my legs through and not get my pants on backwards? Why don't you show me *again,* since I forgot how?"

"Wouldn't you really rather remember how to put your pants on and then use our time together for a story later on?"

I had put on my mother's cap and had no thought for anything but this, my daughter.

"Yes, I suppose." Then Marilyn gazed at me with her velvet brown eyes, the lashes so thick and long, and continued in sweet simplicity. "But I have you right here this minute, and I might not have you to myself later on, when it's story time. You might be off someplace! So I'll take you right now to help me with the pants, since I forgot how."

I caught my breath, for I felt that Marilyn had just slapped me across the face. So it was true, a bird in the hand was worth two in the bush! There had been too many broken promises and too many interruptions. Plans in our family were always made with an *if. If* there is no emergency that calls me away. *If* there is no accident brought into the hospital. *If* there aren't a million phone calls. *If, if, if!* My children couldn't count on a thing and never could I make promises to them. I was hurt, but mostly I was concerned because it had been so easy for this charming, guileless child of mine to slip into the devious cloak of deceit in order to get what she wanted and needed. Her mother.

I fought down the beginnings of a lump in my throat, swallowed quickly and said with a forced smile, "Well, now, you put your own pants on and I won't change my clothes after all. I'll stay right here with you and tell you a story right now, this very moment, while *you* dress *yourself.* . . . Once upon a time . . ." and I started one of my made-up "out of my head" stories, which our children always loved, while Marilyn, memory fully restored, easily finished the rest of her dressing, even to putting on her socks and tying her shoes. The child was three and a half and had just learned to tie a bow. Marilyn had dainty little hesitating fingers which worked at the shoelaces with an awkward grace, and as each bow was made and the loops were given a last tug to tighten them, it was as if her fingers made a small curtsy at the end of a dance.

"Gee, Ma," said Raymond, who was halfway through his breakfast by the time Marilyn and I joined the family. "You didn't change out of your large-animal clothes."

"No, Ray. Marilyn and I needed a little visit and that was more important. All your schoolbooks in order?"

"Yes, Ma. Where did you go this morning, anyway?"

"To the Hansens'."

"I like them. Wish *I* lived on a farm like theirs. Say, can we go swimming in their creek sometime? Mr. Hansen said we should swim there anytime we wanted."

"I don't see why not, when the weather gets warm. I'll pack a picnic lunch." I smiled.

"And *if* there's no 'mergency," piped Marilyn, waving her spoon to emphasize the "if" and accent every word, *"then maybe you'll get to go!"*

"Aw, come off of it, Marilyn. If our own dog, Star, was hit by a car and bleeding and all that, how would you like it if the doctor you took her to said he couldn't tend to her just then because he promised to take his kids swimming?"

"But that's not the same at all. That would be different," and Marilyn patiently tried to explain to her older brother that Star, our German shepherd, was a special dog and really a part of the family. Why, surely she was just as important to the family as, say, Ray himself!

"Yeah, Marilyn, yeah," placated Raymond.

"The only reason Star is so special to you is because she's yours, Marilyn. Every dog is special to its own particular owner. To most anyone else it's just another dog," explained her father.

"Dad's right, Marilyn," I said, and then, "Joe, will you be home tonight for dinner?"

"Yes, but I have a meeting afterwards, so let's *try* to have dinner on time?"

"*If* there's no 'mergency," piped Marilyn, but she quieted

immediately as Ray gave her a disgusted look and a sharp nudge in the ribs.

"I'll try my best," I answered, ignoring the children. I followed Joe to the door and we kissed goodbye.

"You'll love it out," I told him. "It was still kind of cold at four-thirty, but spring is really on its way. It must be quite warm out now—perhaps even over forty degrees. I do wish spring would last longer. When it's springtime I never get tired."

"Well, well!" Joe murmured as he drew me to him and kissed me again, more deliberately. "Save some of your springtime energy for bedtime and I'll help you celebrate the equinox."

We laughed, and as Joe left I reminded him that with such a sendoff and in such a frame of mind, he was bound to have a most successful day.

I looked down at my not-so-white large-animal pants and my loose pullover sweater.

"I've simply got to get out of these clothes," I mumbled.

"Talking to yourself, Ma? That means you're going crazy," teased Raymond, who was the next to leave the house.

"*Going* crazy? Sometimes I think I already am." I kissed him goodbye and Ray left, saying that he simply had to talk to me when he got home from school, that it was very important and that it had to do with baseball—never getting his "ups," or something like that.

Raymond walked down Albany Avenue toward school, and I treated myself to a quiet moment as my gaze lingered on his receding figure. He was in third grade already and growing up at a nice comfortable rate. Raymond had been born with a sunny, happy disposition, yet he was a bit on the quiet side—an intelligent and sensitive boy. He was never bored. He made friends fairly easily and yet he could spend more time alone with all his interesting pastimes than could most children. He was fair and honest in his play and I was pleased to realize that he never carried any grudges. Ray was born with Joe's bones and looks, but I could claim him as mine by his coloring. Fair complexion, rosy cheeks, blue eyes and blond hair. The blue of his eyes would sparkle when he smiled—which he did easily and frequently—and his lids would crinkle together so that his eyes would partly close. He smiled with his mouth partially open and his head tilted slightly to the left, so that his chin would point to his right shoulder.

He had reached Lyle's corner store down the street by now. Crossing Foxhall Avenue, he was out of sight.

I tore up the stairs two at a time to change into fresh clothes for the office. I wondered where the time had gone as, looking at my soiled slacks, I figured it was almost ten years since my mother had sewn them for me. I recalled that day at Cornell when the box arrived containing a supply of white duck trousers Mother had made for me to wear in large-animal clinic and on farm calls in case I ever got to go. The class of veterinary students used to go as a group on farm calls to learn and observe and help treat the animals, but the veterinary college rule was that girls were *not* to go. I wondered if the school policy had ever changed. The trousers my mother made me were still being worn. God, how many times they had been scrubbed and bleached, yet never a split seam! They held so many memories that they were sentimental duds by this time. Everyone called them my large-animal pants and I wryly wondered if they were describing how I looked when I wore them.

I was in a very good mood. I hoped that while I was sterilizing an extra set of instruments and treating the hospitalized animals, I could spend some time with Marilyn. My busy schedule lately had prevented me from being with the child as much as I wished. I enjoyed my family and loved doing things with and for them. Sometimes I wondered how much of this gratified a sense of pleasure, how much a sense of duty. To this day sometimes I can't differentiate the two.

Downstairs again, I found Mame in the kitchen.

"Where did Marilyn disappear to, Mame?"

"Janice was already out in her backyard, and Marilyn asked if she could go next door and play with her. I said sure."

"Darn it! That little monkey made me feel so guilty upstairs before breakfast. I really do not spend enough time with her. Now that I could be with her awhile before office hours, she's off doing something else. I guess she doesn't need me now. I wish, though, for a big fat once, she'd need me when it was *easy* for me to be with her and I wasn't so rushed. Well, I'll ask her if she'd like to be in the office with me for a while, so at least she knows I'd like to be with her."

"No, Mommy," Marilyn replied when I asked her. "I can't come with you now. Janice and I decided that our dolls were going to be sick today and they will need us. Will you be lonesome without me, Mommy?"

"No, Marilyn. I'd just enjoy being with you if you wanted me."

"Well, now! I *always* want you, Mommy. It's just—well, I just don't need you now. I mean, the dolls are very sick and I just *can't* leave."

"Mommy understands," I said, wanting to save the girl from having to make excuses for what were, after all, honest feelings. "I understand exactly how it is to have people who need you when they have someone or something sick."

I could see the flood of relief and look of comradely understanding that bathed Marilyn's face, but then I said something that snapped our thread of rapport.

"Have fun!"

"Fun?" cried Marilyn in disbelief. "These dolls are sick, very sick, and Janice and I will be too busy and worried to have fun." Marilyn bustled, enjoying her responsibilities in a righteously proper way. And suddenly the child's apparent lack of ability to distinguish between pleasure and duty threw new

light on that whole issue. It gave me a new perspective and a fresh sense of proportion. I was sure now that sometimes pleasure and duty are synonymous and this helped explain to me why, when I sometimes was not able to do that which I felt was a pleasure, I sensed guilt. I believe that if it is easy to differentiate a pleasure and a duty, then the duty must be somewhat of a chore. If it is difficult or impossible to differentiate the two, then the duty becomes even more than a pleasure. It becomes a privilege and love makes it a joy.

"Really, Dr. Logue," Mame lectured me as she brought the last of the breakfast coffee into the treatment room. "You shouldn't worry yourself so about not being with Marilyn enough. Why, you spend more time with your kids than most mothers who don't work at all. Honestly, I've worked in homes where I've seen this. And another thing, if you don't mind my saying so: you should be careful and not let those two children of yours know what power they have over you and what an emotional grip they have on you. Kids are quick to catch on and they'll use the power. They'll demand more than is necessary from you and that's not fair to you. Why, I'll bet you're a better wife and mother because you work at this practice, which is something you enjoy, than if you sat at home all day doing nothing and being bored silly."

I set the timer on the sterilizer. "Some women who don't go out of the home to work are completely fulfilled remaining at home, and they don't lack creativity either. Some are marvelous cooks, or expert seamstresses, or terrific gardeners. Now, as far as a family unit is concerned, Mame, don't you really think that's a more ideal situation than our setup?"

"No-o," said the older woman as she thought about it. "Not really. A simpler situation, but not more ideal."

"That's a good way of wording it, Mame. Maybe I ought to simplify things around here—like cutting out evening office hours. Evening hours sure do raise havoc with family life. I often wonder how my husband stands it."

"He stands it," continued Mame, the eternal poor man's philosopher and analyst, "because he loves you. Why, in all the years I've worked in this household I have never heard you two quarrel. You worry too much about neglecting your family, Dr. Logue. Don't massage it so."

"Mm. Perhaps you're right. Anyway," I said with a smile, "thanks for bringing the coffee, Mame, and please be sure to keep a close eye on Marilyn. I'm going to be busy this morning and I won't be able to look out for her myself."

I often wondered how I could run the practice without Mame, for she was more than just a housekeeper; she was a friend who frequently, without being asked, did much more in the line of helpfulness than any housekeeper could ever be ordered to do.

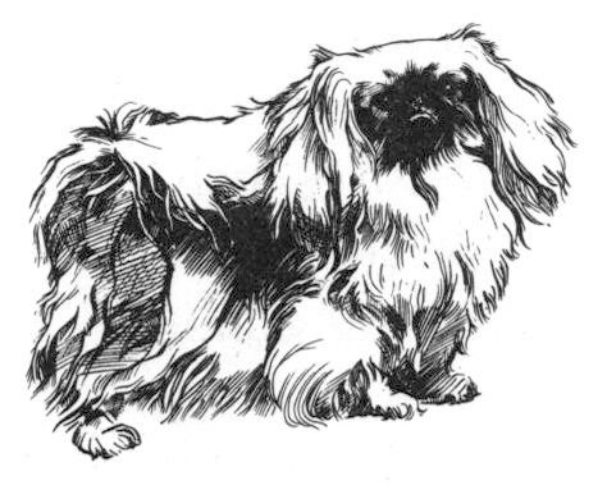

2

I never cease to be amazed and amused by clients' ingenious evasions regarding certain parts of their pet's system that are out of order. If it is an ailment concerning the skin, the eye, the heart, stomach or paw, people speak out in a forthright, uninhibited manner. But let there be a problem with the bowels, the urinary tract or, above all, the genital system, and many people simply cannot discuss it without self-consciousness and discomfort. And the phrases they use to avoid the proper anatomical term!

One afternoon when John, the kennel man, had a free moment, I suggested that he clean the drug closet, wash the shelves and wipe the bottles, being sure to replace each drug in the exact spot where he found it. The drug closet was in a corner of the examining room, and so it was that John was present on the day when Mrs. Wilson entered the room holding her Pekingese out in front of her with such deliberate, meticulous care that you'd think she was carrying the crown jewels. She had phoned me earlier that day about coming, but I couldn't get a word out of her over the phone as to the nature of the dog's problem. It was something the doctor simply *had to see,* was the best I could get in the way of an explanation.

When Mrs. Wilson spied John busy in the drug corner, she abruptly maneuvered her pet so as to tuck its rear end under her arm. Only the Pekingese's pug nose could be seen peeping over the lady's disquieted bosom.

After greeting her pleasantly, I inquired, "What have you noticed about your pet that brings you and Mimi here?"

Mrs. Wilson glanced apprehensively toward John, down protectively at Mimi, and somewhat defensively at me. Then, with another anguished glance at John, she began to whisper. Her back was to John and her free hand went over her mouth so no one could see the words come out. I had a hard time hearing the words as they slipped between the fat fingers of her liver-spotted hands. I remember that she had two rings—one on her index finger and one on her pinky.

"My Mimi—well, my Mimi—I'm worried. I just noticed it, Doctor, just before I phoned you. Mimi has something *hanging"*—this last with great emphasis and one last agonized look at John—"something *hanging* out of her girlie hole!"

I saw John's hand stop in midair. He carefully replaced a bottle of digitalis on the shelf and tiptoed out of the room, his face averted so Mrs. Wilson couldn't see it, for it was red with suppressed laughter, and his lips were contorted into an almost painful grimace as he forcefully confined the peals of laughter which were straining to burst forth. Mrs. Wilson was obviously relieved to be rid of the male animal and I could see that she felt more relaxed now that she could speak to me (a female, thank heavens) privately about the dog's feminine problems. The delicately polite lady finally placed her dog on the table for me to *see.*

Mimi had a pedunculated vaginal polyp—a small tumor that had suddenly popped out through the vulva, where it was dangling like a pink soggy balloon, anchored by about an inch and a half of mucous membrane the diameter of my little finger. The tumor swayed sassily as the Pekingese walked with her pug nose held pretentiously in the air, her plumelike tail carried like a high-fashion ostrich fan.

Over the years there had been many occasions that demanded my control over my facial expressions, so naturally I had more experience than John. Yet I still had to contract my abdominal muscles tightly to quell the incipient quakes of laughter. With a serene and serious face and with what I thought was an impeccable professional attitude, I explained to Mrs. Wilson that this type of tumor was almost always benign and that surgery was the only way to eliminate the dangling appendage. I patiently answered all her questions, explained in detail about the anesthesia, surgery and hospitalization, and all in all spent considerable time with Mrs. Wilson and Mimi.

Then came the classic question asked incredulously by many a pet owner.

"What? I have to *leave* her here?"

The Pekingese was swept off the table into the security of Mrs. Wilson's armpit and the lady retreated with her pet to the waiting room to think it over. All I could see of Mimi, engulfed in her owner's corpulence, was her airy tail and the pink polyp dangling, like an aberrant little tongue panting for air.

(If grownups like Mrs. Wilson were shy about stating their animals' ills, children, on the other hand, were refreshingly candid about it all. I remembered with amusement one time when I was working at the big Manhattan ASPCA hospital when it was still down on Avenue A and East Twenty-fourth Street. A little boy about seven years old waited patiently until it was his turn to see the doctor. He carefully sat his hound, a mixture of all sorts of breeds, on my examining table, and as he wiped his nose on his sleeve, he stated very matter-of-factly, "My dawg can't go to da batroom.")

Mrs. Wilson agonized over whether or not to leave her Mimi with us, but three clients later, she finally returned with her dog to the examining room, anxiety etching the wrinkles on her face into still more deeply creased lines. Little did I know at that moment that this was the beginning of a close association which was to last for years.

"Couldn't you possibly do it right now, Doctor? Mimi won't tolerate being separated from me, you know."

"No, Mrs. Wilson, I cannot do that. Mimi will have to be anesthetized for surgery. She won't miss you while she's asleep, and as soon as I know it's safe, I'll send her home to you. If you could return each day for office treatments, we could shorten her stay in the hospital."

"But are you *absolutely* sure Mimi will be all right?"

"As I explained before, Mrs. Wilson," and I patiently reexplained, "there is always the chance of a problem with any general anesthesia. The surgery itself is not a major undertaking. I'm confident that Mimi will be fine, but I cannot guarantee anything."

Now came the tearful goodbyes, and in no time at all the once poised and snooty Mimi, sensing her owner's fear, was reduced to a shivering, apprehensive animal that snapped in fear at John as he reached to take her from her owner's arms.

"Perhaps Mrs. Wilson would like to put Mimi in the cage herself, John," I quickly suggested. "Mrs. Wilson can see just where little Mimi will be resting while she is with us." What I really wanted to achieve was to keep John with all ten fingers intact, and entirely missing my real point, Mrs. Wilson was pleased by my suggestion and tucked little Mimi into the kennel herself. She watched while John labeled the cage with the name MIMI WILSON and then with another, which read SURGERY. John didn't volunteer to explain that this was really a reminder to himself not to feed the dog the next morning. Mrs. Wilson approved when John gave her pet a pan of water, relaxed when he talked to it kindly for a moment, and was downright gratified when she saw the sign HANDLE GENTLY attached to the cage.

By now Mrs. Wilson had dried her tears, her confidence at least partially restored. An hour and three quarters after she first arrived, she was finally prepared to leave Mimi and go home, repeating several times before she reached the door that she was not going to be able to sleep one wink until her little Mimi was back home with her in her own bed, with her little head on the pillow, the one formerly occupied by her dear deceased husband.

I allowed myself a brief thought as to what Mr. Wilson, looking down from above, perhaps, thought about his replacement. I believed it the better part of discretion not to offer any comment, but I did make a mental note to tell Joe all about it in the evening.

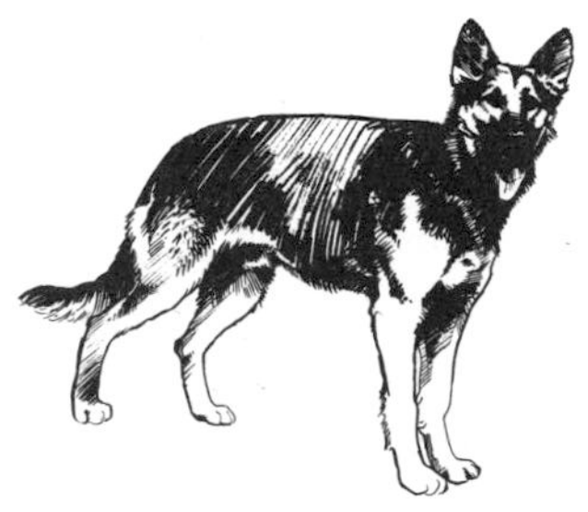

3

A few days later, the weather turned bad. Mame was late and I was preparing breakfast myself. I had broken my right thumbnail down to the flesh the night before, and it felt as if I were opening eggs with a marshmallow. Joe planned to leave for work earlier than usual because of the weather. I planned to leave early also, because I had several farm calls to make, and a lot of driving to do. There were seven-week-old Chester white piglets to be castrated, a dairy herd to be blood-tested for brucellosis and another herd to be tested for tuberculosis. I shuddered to think of all the paper work, all the forms that had to be filled out.

"I know what TB is, of cough," joked Raymond, thinking his pun was tremendously witty, "but what's brucellosis, anyway, Ma?"

"It's an infection that causes abortion or loss of a calf in cattle, and if humans drink unpasteurized milk from an infected cow they can become sick with undulant fever." Joe had answered, seeing that my mouth was full, for I had just taken a big bite from my bacon sandwich and was mopping up my egg yolk with a crust of toast.

"What's castate?" asked Marilyn.

"You mean cast*rate?*" I asked. "Well, there are two glands in male animals which give off something called testosterone.

Now, this testosterone makes the piglet grow into a big strong tough boar which would not be good to make pork chops out of, so we remove these glands when he is a baby. Then the pig grows up and turns out to be not a tough boar, but a tender-muscled animal called a barrow, which is good for eating."

"Was a little pig killed to make this bacon I'm eating?" Marilyn's voice was apprehensive now.

The conversation had taken an unpleasant turn. I wished like anything I could change the subject or even *lie* to Marilyn, but both Joe and I felt strongly that this, in the long run, was the wrong thing to do. We never lied to our children and so I explained the truth as gently as I could.

"Do I have to finish my bacon?" Marilyn pleaded when I finished my explanation, and I made no reply, letting Joe decide what the answer should be. I wasn't passing the buck; I just knew how adamant he was about being a "clean plater." I usually felt that way too, but in this case . . .

I was relieved when Joe tactfully said, "No, Marilyn, you don't have to if you don't want to. I know you like bacon and I suppose you just must feel unusually full this morning and don't have room for it."

"How about me? I don't want to finish my bacon either—it's fatty." Raymond thought he'd latch on to a good thing.

"It's not that bad. Eat it," I said firmly.

"No fair—no fair! Marilyn don't have to eat hers!"

"Raymond . . ." I said slowly, and I reached over and touched his hand, imploring him with my eyes. He darted a glance at his father, who was also staring at him quietly, and suddenly Raymond's resentful expression changed to one of recognition and understanding. He was growing up.

"Oh! Oh, sure! O.K. I *like* bacon!" he said in a manly tone, and both his parents were proud of him.

"Well, I'll just have to go or I'll be late," said Joe, and he put his napkin on the table and rose from his chair. I followed him as usual and we kissed each other goodbye.

"We've got good kids, Jeanne," Joe said.

"Oh, I know it, Joe! And do *you* know what? I love to hear you say it."

I managed to complete three spay operations before I started treating hospitalized animals. Sam, a dog with a broken pelvis and rear leg, was due to go home today and the owners had made arrangements to keep him confined and to restrict his activity. Marilyn had been with me, chatting happily as I snipped and stitched and tied knots. I was glad she seemed no longer upset, and I remembered how Raymond had gone on a vegetarian diet for a short while when he first realized that animals were actually slaughtered in order to provide meat for the table. Joe and I had made no issue of it at the time and gradually he started eating meat again: hot dogs first, then he could tolerate hamburgers, especially if tucked inside a warm roll. The last thing he had accepted was steak, for it must have been a clearer, more obvious reminder of its source.

Mrs. Wilson stopped in unannounced, hoping I could give Mimi a final checkup. She was going to visit her sister, would be gone about a week, and was planning to take the dog along.

"I just want to make sure it's all right for Mimi to travel, Dr. Logue," she called from the waiting room.

"I'll be glad to take a look at her, Mrs. Wilson," I called back to her from the sink, where I was snapping off my surgical gloves. "Come on in to the examining room. I'll be with you in a minute."

In the meantime, Marilyn, a naked doll with a marked lordosis tucked under one arm, took a bottle of alcohol which had a clothes sprinkler on top and proceeded to sprinkle the examining table.

"Mimi is an awful cute dog, Mrs. Wilson," said Marilyn as she started drying the table with a clean towel. Mrs. Wilson heaved her bosom; she was enormously pleased and flattered and just oozed good will, for not only had her Pekingese made an uneventful recovery from her girlie-hole operation, but as an extra dividend, this competent doctor had a charming little girl who liked and admired her pet. Mrs. Wilson doubtlessly figured she had got her money's worth.

When Marilyn slapped her doll face-down on the table and commenced to shove a thermometer into its rubbery behind, Mrs. Wilson tittered and cooed, "What a darling little Florence Nightingale you are, my dear. Tell Mrs. Wilson, dearie, is your dolly sick?"

"Nope." The hand withdrew the thermometer and Marilyn scrutinized it critically. I supposed she was mimicking me.

"Then why are you playing nursie?"

"I'm not playing nursie," Marilyn explained politely, rolling the doll over on its back.

"Well, what are you playing, then?"

"I'm playing *doctor,*" she replied simply as she took a pledget of cotton saturated with alcohol and started to scrub the doll's smooth round rubber belly.

"But what *are* you going to do to her, darling?" persisted Mrs. Wilson with mock solicitude, but mystified nonetheless.

Marilyn paused in her ministrations, looked the lady unwaveringly in the eye, and said in a most professional and precise voice, "I am going to spay her."

I had just finished giving Mimi a clean bill of health and a travel permit, when there was a commotion in the waiting room and an urgent knock on the waiting room door.

A man carrying a large German shepherd and followed by his wife marched in right past Mrs. Wilson and the astonished Mimi. Mrs. Wilson seemed a bit miffed at being so summarily excused.

"Boris came to the side of the bed during the night and woke me. I thought he had terrible gas pains," explained the man.

He had opened his eyes to find their dog resting his chin on the edge of the bed, whining softly. Thinking the animal had to go outdoors, the man had got out of bed and gone to the back door, but Boris hadn't followed. The master returned to the bedroom looking for the dog, and when he turned on the light he saw poor Boris with his back arched in pain, his hind legs extended and stiff.

"I thought he had terrible gas pains," the man said again, "so I tried to coax him to move in hopes it would help him pass the gas and relieve the pressure. He just took a few reluctant steps and gave out. He caved in on the floor with a groan and lay on his right side. I noticed his left side looked swollen, but I thought that was the gas." He blew his nose. He was a short, stocky man with a chest as big as a bourbon barrel. He did not seem to be at all embarrassed by his tears. The Crofts had had Boris since he was a six-week-old pup and had raised all their children with him. The man had over twelve years of memories tied up in the dog. I wasn't embarrassed by the man's tears either. I understood and was most vulnerable to such a poignant situation.

"Well, Ben." It was the first his wife had spoken. She had a soft voice that was compressed by her emotion. She turned to me. "I thought I noticed Boris's abdomen getting gradually bigger, but I only thought he was getting a potbelly because of his age. He's going to be thirteen years old soon."

This was old for a German shepherd.

I questioned Mr. and Mrs. Croft and found that Boris had had transient fainting spells and had become weaker over the past few months. I asked about his appetite, about vomiting, diarrhea or constipation, and was told that his appetite had dropped off considerably, that there had been some vomiting, on and off constipation and lots of gas.

I examined the dog's eyes and mouth and pointed out to them the degree of anemia indicated by the very pale mucous membranes. The dog's abdomen was swollen and bulged on the left side. Just by palpation I could feel an enlarged spleen and I told the owners that Boris might have a splenic tumor. I suggested taking an x-ray to substantiate my tentative diagnosis and I advised an operation.

"Do you think it's cancer, Doctor?" asked Mrs. Croft, fighting down a lump in her throat again as she stroked Boris's ears and head tenderly.

Mr. Croft blew his nose once again. I was sorry I had to tell them the facts.

"To be perfectly honest, there is a high incidence of malignancy in splenic tumors. But let's plan on being lucky; it may turn out to be a benign tumor involving the blood vessels of the spleen. Perhaps it is a torsion or twisting of the spleen. That could cause the severe pain the dog is having, but with the history you have been giving me of how Boris has acted over the past months, I'm skeptical about a torsion. In any event, as to the dog's chances—the prognosis with immediate surgery is decidedly better than no surgery and letting the poor dog remain in pain with a bleeding tumor. He will slowly bleed to death."

And so it was decided that we'd operate. We agreed that if, once the dog was opened, I found that the tumor appeared obviously malignant and had metastasized and spread, and that the dog was inoperable, then I'd give him an overdose of anesthesia to euthanize him.

Mrs. Croft wanted to know what the spleen was for, and how the dog would manage without one. I briefly explained that the spleen stored and concentrated red blood cells, to release them into the bloodstream in time of need—like with a sudden injury and consequent hemorrhage. Filtering the blood as it flowed through the splenic pulp, it removed disintegrating worn-out red cells from the circulation. The iron in these cells was saved and returned to the bone marrow, where it would be incorporated in the production of new red cells. "The third job of the spleen," I continued, "involves not the erythrocytes, or red blood cells, but the leukocytes, or white cells. The spleen produces two types of white cells and is involved in the production of antibodies." I reassured the couple that while the spleen was an important organ, it was not absolutely essential to the continuation of life, and that most of its functions could be taken over by other tissues.

Later, when the surgery was almost over, it looked as if we were all in luck, for I felt sure Boris had just a hemangioma—a benign tumor of the blood vessels—but we could not be certain until I received a report from the pathology lab. I very carefully removed the hugely swollen spleen from the abdominal cavity, taking care not to injure the tail of the pancreas or the greater curvature of the stomach. I completed tying off the fifty-second blood vessel of the spleen. Each blood vessel had double ligatures and each ligature had three knots.

My fingers were tired. I had ligated every blood vessel individually and had tied the ligatures several millimeters from the ends of the severed vessels so as to prevent slippage of the ligatures from the ends of the stumps. I removed hemostats carefully, and just prior to closing the abdomen, inspected every ligature for any sign of bleeding which might possibly lead to postoperative hemorrhage. I did everything possible within the limits of my knowledge to prevent complications following surgery. Surgery takes much *unhurried* time.

The dog's pulse seemed good and all the ligatures were beating a little rhythm as the arterial stumps pulsated like throbbing rubies. The removed spleen had already started turning blue, and it looked like a withering eggplant by the time I placed it on a nearby tray.

"Don't toss that out yet, John. I'll have to check with the owners to see if they want me to send it to the pathology lab to be checked for malignancy. While I finish sewing Boris up, go fetch the second donor dog from the back kennel. I want to continue transfusing Boris with fresh blood."

"Can't you use the bottle of blood you have stored in the refrigerator, Dr. Logue?" John was removing his surgical gloves. When I had first opened Boris and started lifting out his spleen, I discovered that it was larger than I'd expected. I had called out to John to drop everything, scrub up, put on clean gloves and help me, for I needed someone to support the heavy spleen during surgery lest its sagging weight alone might snap and rupture the blood vessels involved.

John had done very well and he appeared to be feeling rather important as he removed the rubber surgical gloves. He was a good kennel man and I wished desperately to keep him. I tried whenever possible to give him tasks that had more interest and responsibility, hoping that he'd be happy with his job and not become fed up with the routine dirty work or the more earthy aspects of his duties. I did not believe in ever being too busy to explain things to him.

"That would be satisfactory," I explained, "if I wished only to replace blood volume, as in shock, but we need platelets now. Platelets are necessary for the clotting process. Fresh blood has functional platelets, while the platelets in stored blood are dead and are useless as far as clotting is concerned."

I had finished putting Boris back together by the time John brought the second donor dog in. The first blood donor, used earlier that morning, had been a huge Great Dane. I fed and treated this dog well, for I never ceased to marvel at the way he conducted himself during a bloodletting. The Dane had been through it many times and seemed to know what was expected. He was large enough so that I could use the radial vein, and the dog would lie obediently on the floor on his abdomen, hind legs tucked up under him, forelegs lying straight out in front of him, like a canine sphinx. John would hold off the vein and I would collect a pint of blood in a vacuum flask that contained an anticoagulant. The whole procedure was pretty much the same as that in a human blood bank. The Great Dane would just sit there quietly, his huge head held nobly erect. He would occasionally bend his neck and look down on the procedure in a tolerant, benevolent manner.

The second donor dog was given a short-acting anesthesia, because the animal was much smaller than the first donor and I had to collect the blood directly from its heart.

Together John and I carried Boris into a large cage in the recovery room. The flask of blood was attached to the top of the cage door and the blood continued to drip down through the tubing into the sleeping dog's vein. I injected penicillin into Boris's buttock, thankful that the price had plummeted in the past few years, to a point where I could afford to use it. It was still expensive and I could not afford to use it routinely, but I figured that Boris, without a spleen to manufacture antibodies and white cells, needed all the help he could get to combat infection postoperatively.

"Mame!" I called down the basement stairs from the kitchen. "Just as soon as you come up from the laundry, will you phone the Crofts? Tell them that the operation is over and their dog is doing as well as can be expected. Ask them if they want the specimen sent to the pathology lab. Tell them Boris had a tumor and it looks like a benign one, but I can't be sure without pathology work being done. Tell them they can phone me tonight around eight-thirty if they want to. We won't contact them unless we have bad news."

I checked the German shepherd once more, and seeing that there was nothing further to be done for him at the time, I prepared to treat hospital cases. Mame came in to get the Crofts' number, and I heard her ask the operator for 297. She gave my message to Mrs. Croft, then I heard her say, "Just a moment," and the next thing I knew, Mame was by my side in the examining room.

"Mrs. Croft wonders if she could talk to you."

"Please tell her I can't come to the phone right now," I answered as I worked. "I don't mean to be short with her, Mame, but there's really nothing further to discuss with her. I spent a lot of time explaining everything earlier this morning. You might tell her again, though, that if she wants me to send the spleen to the lab I'll be glad to and that I can give further news about Boris if they phone after eight-thirty tonight."

"I understand, Dr. Logue. I'll tell them to phone you tonight and that the dog is fine."

"No, no! Don't tell them that, Mame. Just say he's doing as well as can be expected. To say he's fine may give them false confidence. Things could take a turn for the worse. The dog can still go into shock and die. Just say his condition is satisfactory."

I finally got around to treating the pets of the people who were waiting in the office. I was terribly behind schedule because of Boris, the unscheduled happening, and I wondered at the patience of those pet owners and whether I'd have the patience to sit for almost an hour if our roles were reversed.

The first patient was a wounded cat. An alert young woman dressed in a pullover sweater and slacks held her pet while I treated it. The phone rang and John answered, then relayed the message that a man had a lame horse and wanted a doctor.

I let out a groan and did some mental calculations. I still had to finish with all the people in the office and then I had to get to a dairy herd to check the results of the intradermal tuberculin I had injected three days before. The requisite seventy-two hours were up today. Then there was the routine surgery I hadn't had time for that morning because of Boris.

There were three appointments for late afternoon. Then there was grabbing dinner before evening office hours.

"John, tell him the very earliest I could get there would be nine or ten tonight or tomorrow morning and that I suggest he call another vet. Tell him I'm sorry, but I can't make it any sooner."

John conveyed the message while I treated the cat's wound. The animal was not a bit appreciative and both the owner, holding the cat, and I had to pay attention not to get clawed or bitten.

"He says the horse has been lame for three days and that it's real bad today."

I looked at my client and rolled my eyes ceilingward. I suppose it was unprofessional, but I was beginning not to give a damn, so I blurted out, "Oh, great! If I dropped *everything* right now to go to him, I'd still probably get there in time to witness the horse dying from a fulminating septicemia. Well, I'm sorrier than ever, but the length of time his horse has been lame doesn't alter my packed schedule one iota. I *still* cannot get there before late tonight. Considering how long the horse has been lame, though, stress how important it is for him to get someone else sooner! I just can't put off routine surgery again today."

John talked into the telephone again and suddenly jerked the receiver away from his ear. The young lady clutching her cat kept turning her head from John to me and back to John again, intent on every word of our conversation. We could both hear a loud noise coming from the phone all the way across the room, though we couldn't make out the words.

John suddenly, without one more word, slammed down the receiver in an angry, indignant gesture.

"John!" I admonished. "What's the matter? That wasn't very polite." I flushed the cat's wound with hydrogen peroxide and it bubbled and foamed like a frothing glass of beer.

"Boy, was he mad!" exclaimed John. "He bawled something about trying to get a vet when you needed one and then he said he's already called all the others and that you were the last on his list."

I wasn't exactly flattered by this, yet I decided a magnanimous tolerance was the most dignified course for me to take, so I mopped the cat's foaming brew and said, "So why get all upset and hang up on him?"

"Well, he also said—er—well—" and John looked uncomfortable and lapsed into an embarrassed silence.

"Suppose we discuss it later, John." My hands continued to heal the sick.

"No, Dr. Logue! *Please?"* interjected the young pet owner. Her eyes were alight with a feverish gleam, so eager was she for a bit of gossip.

"Please? That man! What did he say?" she asked with an imploring expectancy. I decided that since she had patiently endured the long wait for me in the outer room, she was entitled to some compensation, so after pausing a moment I said, "All right, John. All right. Out with it. Tell us, what *did* he say?"

"Well, he said you were last on his list to call and he figured maybe you wouldn't be so busy and could come because nobody much would bother to call you since you're just a—just a—" John looked miserably uncomfortable and stared at the frothy mess on the table.

"Just a *what?*" both client and I demanded of him in the same breath.

"A dumb broad! That's what he called you, Doctor, a dumb broad!"

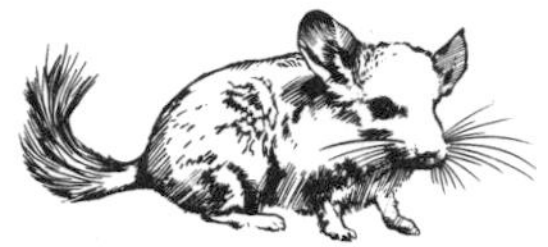

4

All too quickly, it seemed, the time came for Marilyn to enter kindergarten. She had been very excited about starting school and threw herself into the social whirl with bright-eyed enthusiasm.

Marilyn had Joe's coloring and features. Her hair had a slight tendency to curl and an unusually high sheen. I have never seen anything so wet-looking in its shine, yet in actuality so fluffy dry. She was almost always smiling, and in doing so, held her head straight with her chin tucked under slightly. There was a trace of a dimple in her left cheek, which looked as if it would disappear as she grew older. While her brother made friends easily, Marilyn made them very easily, and I was sure she'd grow up to become a social director of some kind. She was most content when she felt she had helped make someone happy. With her sunny disposition, dancing eyes and rosy cheeks, Marilyn always reminded me of Samuel Taylor Coleridge's poem:

> A little child, a limber elf,
> Singing, dancing to itself,
> A fairy thing with round red cheeks,
> That always finds and never seeks.

For all this, my daughter still had some pretty profound moments. Her chief concern was that the family always seemed too busy. On the few occasions that the four of us planned to go on a picnic or to a drive-in movie, it was Marilyn who would be out in the driveway first, standing next to the car, frantically hopping on one leg and then the other, in a restless urgency to get going.

"Hurry, Mother! Hurry, before someone comes with an animal and we can't go."

Both children did have to cope with too many broken promises.

Marilyn confided in me one bedtime when I was tucking her in that when she grew up and got married, she was going to arrange things so that her family would not be too busy.

"I'm going to see to it that everybody takes time to enjoy one another," was the way she put it. I felt very close to Marilyn then. I fleetingly, but oh, so clearly, recalled my father's weary attitude toward the passage of his days and my own high resolve as a child to make a different way of life when my time came.

I missed Marilyn in the office and my clients missed her too, for Marilyn just oozed love. Even some of the tougher male clients succumbed to her charm. She dripped with concern for all their animals and the owners lapped it up. It must have given them a sense of well-being, for they assumed (and they assumed correctly) that the child's sincere and genuine interest in their pets' welfare was an extension of her mother's concern.

One thing Marilyn and I never forgot was that each person leaving a sick animal with us thought his case just a little more urgent, more out of the ordinary; to him nothing was ever routine, and most of all, his pet was always very, very special.

Sometimes I'd wish that the practice wouldn't keep growing

so. I kind of wanted to keep the status quo and not risk developing "bigness disease," where animals just come and go, and each case is just another file card. Yet I realized that a business or profession or any venture that stands still very long is in a sense slipping backward. Somehow things always seem to have to enlarge, expand and progress. Progress or go backward, I had concluded long ago.

There is no such thing as standing still.

I had hired John's wife, Debbie, to take care of the office, acting as a receptionist, answering the phone and doing some filing. Debbie's mother had offered to take care of their little girl, two and a half years old, and it seemed to be a tidy answer to my need for more help and John's need for extra family income.

I had already given up making house calls for small animals; there simply were no longer enough hours in the day for such calls. This helped to smooth the daily routine, but hardly scratched the surface as far as really relieving the work load. I decided I needed a second veterinarian and began to make plans to interview veterinary students who were to graduate from college in June.

"I'll develop these x-rays for you, Dr. Logue," Mame volunteered as she brought a fresh pot of coffee into the office for Debbie, John and me to share. Since Marilyn had started school, Mame had spent an increasing amount of time helping in the office. Without being asked, she had started taking such things as ironing and mending home with her to do in the evening. I was very touched by Mame's dedication and thoughtfulness, for I needed and truly appreciated the extra help in the office.

John came from the hospital's recovery room into the examining room, carrying the next patient in a small cardboard carton. Mame had just emerged from the darkroom. The pictures were all developed and were hanging on the racks to dry.

"What in heaven's name is that?" queried Mame as she saw the tiny creature in the box.

"Feel it and guess!" I suggested. Both Mame and John knew it was not a mouse or a rat or a hamster; they wouldn't even venture to guess what it was.

"Doesn't the fur give you a clue? They make coats out of these. May I introduce *Chinchilla laniger,* and would you believe that I did a Caesarean section on her last night?"

"Well, now I've seen everything!" Debbie exclaimed. "What nut would spend good money for an operation on a ratty-looking little thing like that?"

"Its owners would. They own a chinchilla farm and this is their best breeding female. Do you have any idea of the value of a good breeding pair of chinchillas?"

"No, and I'll tell you this—I wouldn't give you a nickel for them!" the girl answered, refusing to touch the creature when I held it out to her so that she could feel the luxuriant thickness and breath-taking softness of the fur.

"Well, I was flabbergasted to learn that a good breeding pair will bring as much as three thousand dollars. This one is half of a prize-winning pair and the owners will go to great lengths to save her."

Debbie was beginning to exasperate me. She was lazy and vain, and somewhat less than interested in the activities of the office.

I turned the chinchilla on its back to examine the tiny incision. It was dry and the skin was nicely approximated; so far, I was satisfied with the chinchilla's progress. The uterus was so very tiny and the two fetuses I had found inside, one dead and one alive, had been curled like little rounded silver lima beans. The mother had delivered three normal young ones on her own and had acted normal until about fourteen hours later, when she became lethargic and no longer paid attention to her young. The owners had brought her in to me the evening before, and after the cause of the trouble was discovered (the diagnostic instrument being the tip of my little finger) I found myself unable to extract the dead fetus. I had suggested a Caesarean as a last resort. I told them that without the surgery the chinchilla would die and I added very frankly that I had never operated on a chinchilla before and had never seen a description of the procedure in the medical journals. I could only be guided by judgment gained from experience with other animals. The information I needed was not to be learned from books. Who's to know, until it's tried, the safest type of anesthesia for a chinchilla? Who's to know what drugs this species will tolerate or what the exact dosage should be? I explained to the owner the curious fact that morphine is a depressant for dogs but that its action on the cat is just the opposite—domestic cats, lions, tigers, all are stimulated by morphine. They'll run about the room, make all manner of circus movements, and even attempt to climb the walls. They make no effort to escape if chased and don't even try to avoid obstacles as do normal animals. But the first man to give a cat morphine couldn't know what was going to happen; since morphine is a depressant for most animals, he could only assume it would also depress a cat.

"I'm beginning to get your message," the owner of the chinchilla had commented, rubbing his jaw in contemplation. "I guess I have everything to gain and nothing to lose, so go ahead and operate."

After weighing all the pros and cons, I used gas to anesthetize the little animal so that I could regulate the depth of anesthesia more readily. Even though it was a general anesthesia and I might lose the one baby left inside, it was safest for the mother, and it was this fact that influenced my decision.

I tucked the entire chinchilla into the ether cone, and after a short struggle during which she tried to get out, she finally ceased moving and fell asleep. From that moment on, I was a one-man band, for I soon discovered that the margin of surgical anesthesia was *very* narrow. The chinchilla was either too deeply asleep or too lightly so. She was constantly either on the verge of regaining consciousness or on the verge of dying. Once the tiny creature stopped breathing and I had to stop the operation completely so I could administer artificial respiration. I thought surely I had lost her, but with painstaking effort and in an agony of worry, I kept pinching that fragile rib cage in and out, and the game little thing started breathing for me again. I no sooner got the second baby out—the one that by some miracle was still alive after all this—when, by gum, the mother started shivering and regaining consciousness. Quickly I had to pop her into the cone again, a pledget of cotton saturated with the anesthetic near her nose. And so it went, but finally the operation was finished, with the one baby and the mother alive.

I must admit that I felt a wholesome sense of satisfaction as I watched the mother chinchilla wash her tiny infant. Now I was qualified to write a report on chinchilla surgery for the medical journals. All I needed was the time!

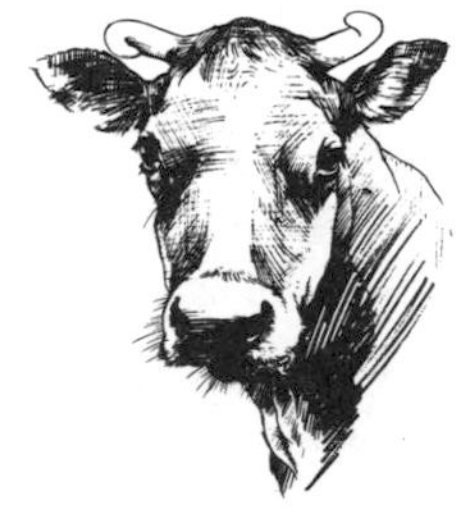

5

One bitter-cold morning, by amazing coincidence, I had two cows in a row with the same problem. It all started with an urgent call to treat a newborn calf overcome with scours, a neonatal diarrhea that can kill very quickly. I had just finished treating the calf when its owner, Mr. Schmidt, became apoplectic. His eyes grew large and then almost popped out of their sockets and rested on his cheeks as he let out a yell.

"Gott! Doctor, Doctor! Come *quick!*"

He was glued to the floor of the barn, two stalls down, his pop eyes staring at the cow lying there.

"If you think Mr. Schmidt's eyes were popped," I said to Joe later that day, "you should have seen that cow's uterus. *Popped completely out* of the cow!"

There the poor thing lay with what looked like a huge dirty laundry bag hanging from her rear. The uterus, still moist and warm from just being inside the cow, was steaming. It quivered and then flowed still further over the cold barn floor.

All of my old teacher Dr. Dank's lecture on the prolapsed uterus came flooding back to me; I have a good auditory memory. "Do this . . . do that . . . inject posterior pituitary extract . . . Pitocin . . ." I could hear and see him now, intelligent, quick and decisive.

"Shall I call the butcher?" This from Schmidt.

"Lots of warm water!" I bawled, and waved my arm like an army sergeant.

While he was on his errand, I injected Dr. Dank's recommended hormone into the cow's rump muscle. PITUITARY OXYTOCIC PRINCIPLE—POP, the little vial was labeled, an altogether fitting name for this drug, I thought, considering what the cow's uterus had done. I never saw anything work so wonderfully fast. I must have hit a blood vessel to get such swift results. That uterus gave one shudder and literally popped right back inside the cow! The whole maneuver gave the impression of a large mouth sucking back the hugest bubble gum bubble I ever saw. *Shloop!* It was gone!

The farmer returned, and his eyes, back in their sockets by now, popped out all over again.

"Where did it go?" He looked around in bewilderment as if the thing might have crawled away on its own and sequestered itself in some dark corner.

I dried my hands and started methodically to roll down my sleeves.

"I fixed it."

"But—but what will I do with all this hot water?"

"Gosh, I don't know, Mr. Schmidt. Do you have any tea bags around?"

Mr. Schmidt was ecstatic. He called all his hired hands, and a sudden assortment of overalls in various degrees of faded blue were standing around me, admiring me as if I were a movie star.

I adored every minute of it.

I showed the men how to make an elevated wooden ramp for the cow to stand on to elevate her rear end. Gravity would cause the uterus to slide forward in her body and help prevent a recurrence of the prolapse. It reminded me of the knee-chest position my doctor had suggested I assume for fifteen minutes a day after my babies were born, to slide my organs back into place. I figured if it was good enough for me, it was good enough for a cow.

The farmer's wife interrupted the accolades. I had been intercepted by a phone call. It seems a cow had just been discovered with her insides on the barn floor. Another prolapse!

I hurried to take my leave. Someone slapped me on the shoulder and said, "By gar! They have the right vooman for the chob."

Someone else opened the door of my chariot for me, I was helped into my seat and the door was closed. I drove off, leaving my fans behind, smiling and waving goodbye.

I drove along full of confidence and feeling pretty pleased with myself. I figured I had this next case made.

There was the uterus, on the floor. This one was not steaming. It was cold, drying out somewhat and looking slightly leathery, like someone's discarded satchel.

I tried for over two hours to replace that cow's uterus. I kneaded the organ with bath towels dripping with hot water, hot as my hands could stand. The uterus was steaming now, along with the towels. So were my hands. They were red and swollen, hot and steaming, while the rest of me was freezing.

Three young children stood in a row, watching me. It was a serious occasion: they had missed the school bus and still they looked sad. Their mother and father watched too, also in tight-lipped solemnity. The children's shoes were worn and shabby and their clothes showed signs of frequent patchings. Obviously they were a poor family and this was their only cow. I turned to the beast in desperation. I *must* save this cow for them. I *must.*

I tried once more. In spite of all my efforts, my hot compresses and my magical POP, the uterus didn't give even a ripple. It remained lying in my lap, flaccid.

I sighed. "Call the butcher."

I felt so bad for this family and their cow. I was suddenly ashamed of my conceited glory of a few hours before. I couldn't bear to look into the children's faces and I fought back a lump of remorse which was rising in my throat.

I crawled over to my bags and packed them and then forcefully straightened my cramped back and knees.

"How much do I owe you, Doc?" asked the head of the family. He reached toward his frayed jeans pocket.

The independent, small-operation farmer—the backbone of America, I thought to myself. Poor, but honest . . . poor but honest.

I looked at his children now. I wanted to gather all three ragamuffins to my bosom. I wanted to take them all home with me and love them. I didn't want to take their father's money, but I mustn't hurt his pride.

"Five dollars?" I said timidly, and then I blurted out, "Oh, I'm so sorry, Mr. Johnson, so awfully, awfully sorry."

He patted my shoulder gently and said in the kindest voice I ever heard, "Now, don't you feel so bad about this. You done the very best you could."

I felt worse than ever. This man was *kind* and poor but honest.

He put his hand into a back pocket and pulled out a fistful of green bills. Then he put his other hand into another back pocket and pulled out another fistful. My eyes popped as I watched them unfurl. The snarl of green bills expanded and grew in his hands like fast-growing heads of green cabbage. Tens and twenties and even fifties! I never saw so much money in my life! It was difficult for him to find so small a denomination as five dollars, but the poor honest man persevered in his search and was finally successful, and he duly paid me my fee.

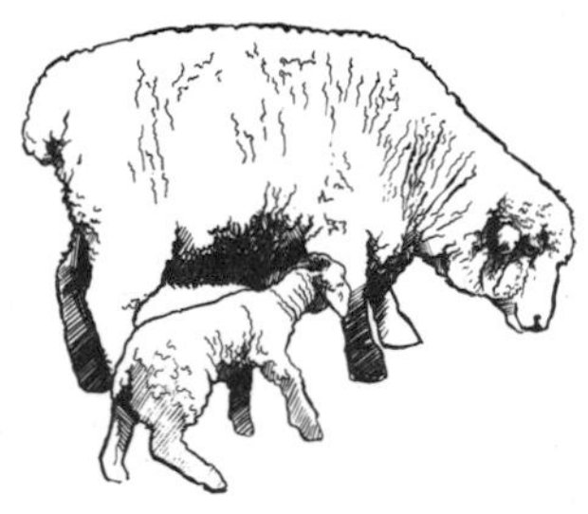

6

It was Labor Day weekend, 1952, and that year the annual Labor Day picnic was to be held at our place. There were four couples, old friends, who took turns hosting the picnic each year, and while the reunions were always unpretentious, very informal affairs, they were a highlight of the year for everyone involved. Each visiting couple brought something—a salad, baked beans, or a dessert, and the host couple always supplied the keg of beer, the clams and the mainstay of the meal, usually steak or lobster. The annual picnics had been started by the Munroes years ago, when Raymond was about four years old. One couple, the Morgans, had come from some distance for this year's reunion and they were staying with us for the weekend. The Munroes and the Sentells lived close enough so that they could easily make the picnic in one day. We all knew each other well enough so that if I was called away on a case during the day, all the girls would take over with the preparations and the festivities could go on without interruption.

I was especially enjoying preparing breakfast for the Logues and the Morgans this Labor Day morning, and I wanted to make it a holiday affair. Finally breakfast was ready and everyone gathered about the breakfast table. We had just started the meal when the phone rang.

"Dr. Logue speaking," I said.

"Dr. Logue, this is Nate Adams."

"Yes, Nate."

"I'm sorry to bother you on a holiday, but I just noticed one of my ewes. She must be sick because she's lagging behind the flock and standing alone."

"Do you have any idea if she's still eating?" I inquired.

"To tell you the truth, I don't." Nate's voice sounded apologetic. "We just feed them and they all eat together and graze together."

"Is this the first day you noticed the ewe alone?"

"Yes, ma'am. Just last night and this morning."

"Has she ever lambed?"

"Yes. She was bred the beginning of last November and lambed last spring, in March."

"Was everything O.K.? Was there ever any discharge?"

"No. I never noticed anything. At lambing time everything seemed normal."

I knew, as Nate did, that sheep are social animals, needing the close company of the other sheep in the flock in order to function normally. If any sheep separated itself from the flock, it was a bad sign, like the tail of a sick pig which has lost its curl. Crude diagnostic methods, perhaps, but nonetheless reliable. I knew that Nate ran a first-rate Shropshire sheep farm. He probably knew about as much concerning sheep as I did, give or take a few medical technicalities, and if Nate was asking for help, he really needed it.

"I'll be right there, Nate. Just let me gather my gear together."

I explained matters to the folks in the dining room.

"Jesus H. Christ!" Joe exploded, and children's faces turned to him in surprise. "Can't it wait until later? Sit down, for Christ's sake, and eat breakfast!"

"I can't enjoy it now, Joe. I'll be back just as soon as I can."

Mary Morgan quickly said, "I'll make sure all the children are fed, Jeanne, and I'll clean up the kitchen—so relax." And she wiped her youngsters' fingers, sticky with raspberry jam. "I'll keep a pot of coffee on for you so you can have a cup when you get back. Never you mind, now; I'll tend the store while you're gone. I'll get Joe and Bob to start cooling the keg of beer."

I thanked Mary, and Joe followed me into the office.

"Jeanne," he said, "you're wrong. Dead wrong. There's no reason why we can't all sit down like human beings for once and have an uninterrupted, leisurely breakfast. I'm sorry I didn't take the phone off the hook! For us to all eat together would take at most half an hour. One lousy half hour. If the animal can't last half an hour longer, it isn't going to live anyway."

"Yes, Joe, I know what you mean, sweetie, but don't you understand? I just can't relax and eat a leisurely meal and chat and talk over coffee when to my mind that lousy half hour might make all the difference in the world. I simply can't do it! If I could, I ought to take down my shingle. Can't you understand?"

"Forget it, Jeanne. Just forget this whole conversation." And he pecked me a kiss goodbye.

I followed Nate to the barnyard, where he showed me the sick ewe.

"She lagged behind last night when the rest of the sheep came in. This morning when the flock was let out, she didn't go with them. She just stood here alone in the barnyard."

I walked slowly and quietly over to the docile animal, rubbed its head and felt its ears. I took the animal's temperature while it was still quiet and not alarmed or aroused by my examination. The thermometer read a low normal and next I checked the oral mucous membranes, the nose, the eyes, the heart and the lungs. Her membranes seemed a little paler than normal, but other than that, there was nothing unusual.

"You say she had a lamb last spring. Was there anything at all unusual about the lambing?" Puzzled, I repeated the question I had put to him over the phone.

"No," said Nate positively. "She was fine and has been, to my knowledge, until last night."

I felt the animal all over and remarked about the extreme emaciation I found.

"Just feel her, Nate! She's skin and bones." And I started palpating the sheep's abdomen. My hand bumped against something hard. I felt again.

"Maybe she has an abdominal tumor—possibly a firm fibrous mass." I thought aloud so Nate could hear. "I'm stumped, Nate. It could be a tumor or a walled-off abscess. She almost looks toxic to me and yet the temperature is normal. Of course, she could have been running a fever for some time, and who would know? We might just be catching this temperature reading just as it's beginning to fall. It may be on its way down to a subnormal level and just by coincidence we may have caught it while it's still within normal limits. A heavily parasitized animal could look like this. . . ." I continued to cast about in my mind. "I have a feeling she's sicker than we think. I could fit her in the rear of the station wagon and take her back to the hospital with me. It would help to know what some lab work would turn up and I'd like to take an abdominal x-ray of that mass I felt. Honestly, Nate, I hate to say it, but deep down, I feel this ewe might die."

"I think so too, Dr. Logue," agreed the veteran sheepman. "I'll tell you what. In this business, it's all a question of economics. I like the animals and all that, but I can't afford to go overboard as far as money is concerned just to try to save one ewe. Let's just do the blood and urine tests and skip the hospitalization. In the meantime, do what you can for her.

Let's give her one more day and if it still looks like a lost cause, we'll just put her down. It's the best I can afford to do."

"O.K., Nate, but if things go wrong, can I have her for autopsy? It won't cost you anything and I'm sure we'll both learn something."

"All right, Dr. Logue. It's a deal," said Nate, nodding his head in agreement, and so I collected some blood and some urine, gave the animal supportive treatment, and promised Nate that I'd let him know what I found after the lab work was done.

"But you know, Doc . . ." Nate pursued the issue, scratching his head in perplexity. "About your thinking this ewe might be toxic . . . I don't think that's it. If it was poisoning, some of the others ought to show signs. That flock of sheep has always been together and none of the others are sick."

"I understand, Nate, but I was thinking more along the line of being toxic from an infection or an autointoxication—a self-poisoning, you know?"

"It beats me, Doc. I never saw an animal like this one before."

By the time I returned home, everyone was there. The fellows had the keg of beer cooling on ice and they were rinsing off the clams. While I had some coffee, we women exchanged news and items of interest, mainly concerning our husbands and children. We had a lot of catching up to do and there was much lively chatter. It was a happy reunion.

We joined the men outdoors and since lunchtime was approaching, I suggested to Joe that he get the charcoal started. Hot dogs and hamburgers were for lunch; the lobster we had on hand was for our dinner. There was much good-natured joking and eventually the talk got around to politics. It always did.

"The government had better start tightening its belt—now,"

Joe expounded. "If we keep this up, in twenty years the United States will go broke. Spend, spend, spend—and pass laws. Slap one law on top of another and spend—rob Peter to pay Paul—That's all those politicians know how to do—"

"Someone give a yell when the charcoal is covered with a gray ash and we're ready to start cooking," I said. The women and I were carrying platters of food from the kitchen and had already set the picnic tables, all the while continuing to interject into the discussion our opinions, participating just as noisily but perhaps not so blasphemously as the men.

The fellows offered to grill the meat and the girls volunteered to start feeding all the children, while I left to treat the necessary cases in the hospital. Raymond and the Munroe boy helped me hold the animals as I treated them and together we fed them all and gave them fresh water. It was John's day off, and after the boys returned to the picnic and I had a moment to myself, I ran through the urinanalysis and did some blood chemistry on Nate Adams's ewe.

Since sheep are herbivorous animals, I expected to find the urine alkaline, but to my surprise, it was strongly acid in its reaction. Though this could be accounted for in an animal with a high-protein diet, like meat, it was an unlikely situation in an animal eating only vegetation. There was also a four-plus albumen, which could be due to various causes—one of them being toxicity. The sheep's white cell count was very high, as in cases of infection.

I gave a sigh of frustration, for I still lacked enough information to be sure of any diagnosis, but I did believe more strongly than ever that we were dealing with either the tail end of a general debilitating infection or an intoxication of some kind. I just had a feeling that the ewe's temperature would continue to fall and that the correct diagnosis would be made when I did an autopsy.

I rejoined the crowd. Joe brought me a hamburger he had

kept warm for me and garnished with a slice of Italian onion, crisp and white, with concentric colorful rings of its purple-blue skin. On top of this was swirled some pickle relish, and with a flourish came a snarl of mustard.

"*Et voilà!*" and he gave the creation to me with a mug of cold beer and a kiss that conveyed a happier message than the petulant peck I had received from him when I left for Nate Adams's earlier in the day.

I phoned Nate early the next morning and he reported that the ewe was about the same, maybe a little quieter, and would neither eat nor drink. The news didn't surprise me, and I in turn conveyed the results of the lab work, and my interpretation of them. It was agreed that the ewe was to be euthanized and I planned to leave for Nate's farm as soon as I finished treating hospital cases.

Later in the day, as I walked from my car to the barnyard, I saw Nate in the distance, standing next to the doomed animal, looking down at her. The man had a good "sheep personality," I decided, for there was a passivity of disposition, a shyness and a quiet, slow deliberateness of motion about Nate which were much like the behavior patterns of the very sheep he tended. In fact, even Nate's hair looked a little like a sheep's. It had turned a snowy white, and his skull and finely wrinkled face appeared to have been tucked snugly into a tightly curled woolly winter cap. He had rather small, but bright, brown eyes which blinked infrequently and rather slowly, and his eyebrows, also white, had grown bushier and longer with old age. While the hair on Nate's head reminded me of the wool found on the Merino or Rambouillet, two fine-wool breeds of sheep, his eyebrows distinctly had an Angora texture; they were so long and silky.

The little ewe standing meekly by his side was a Shropshire, a mutton-type breed, and she was apathetic and submissive now, almost to the point of being oblivious of my ministrations. I checked her temperature; it had indeed gone down, for the thermometer barely registered a chilly ninety-seven degrees.

Nate steadied the animal and held its unresisting soft fleecy head in his arms as I injected a concentrated solution of sodium pentobarbital into the ewe's jugular vien. Before the needle was withdrawn, the ewe, innocent of the fact that she was being killed, was dead. She lay on the ground like a piece of tumbleweed made all of white cotton, and a sudden soft gust of warm wind blew on her, stirring her wool. It rippled just as grass is rippled by the wind as it blows by.

Upon opening and exploring the ewe, I found that the animal, unknown to anyone, had been carrying twin lambs that previous spring, and from the looks of things, had carried both lambs to full term. One lamb had been born normally and uneventfully; the second lamb was never born. Why? No one could know the answer. The ewe had carried the dead lamb within her the remainder of that spring and all summer long, and nature valiantly had tried to make things right again, for the mother's body had almost succeeded in reabsorbing the entire lamb's body through her own system. Indeed, all that remained of that unborn lamb now was a disconnected mass of bones and a few tufts of hair, all floating in a black soupy exudate within the uterus. I stared in silence, for I was humbled by this magnificent effort expended by a living organism to rid itself of a toxic body. The wonder of it all.

When I thought of all the complex protein molecules which had been broken down and reduced to their basic ions and then excreted through the mother's system, I was impressed all over again. Muscles, ligaments, tendons, all soft tissue except a few tufts of hair, were gone! Even the cloven hoofs, tiny foot bones and part of the lower jaw had been reabsorbed.

I placed the bones and tufts of hair carefully on a white

towel. The bones were black and looked charred, dull sticks of unpolished raw ebony against the white background where they lay like prehistoric relics taken from some ancient tomb.

The results of the lab work made sense now. The acid urine, seen in animals with a high protein intake? Of course the ewe had a high protein intake! Had she not been digesting a fully developed lamb all summer? The urine test with the four-plus albumen? This made sense now too. No wonder when I first saw the ewe I thought she might be toxic—and no wonder the white cell count had been so high and the blood urea nitrogen so far above normal.

All the pieces of the puzzle fit into place now, and oh, to think of it! Nature almost succeeded too!

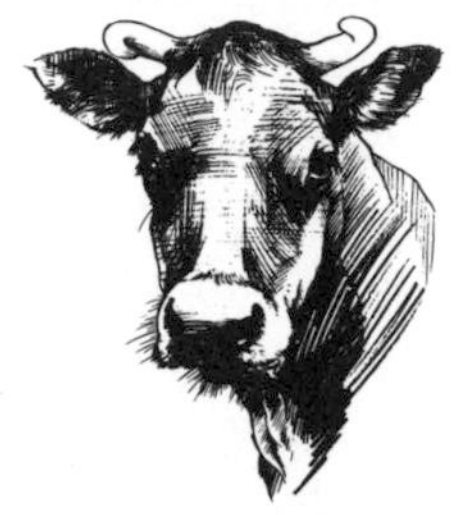

7

The lake was a sheet of silver under the moonlit sky. The more timid stars had shyly faded away, and others were to be found cringing as if in awe of the moon's brilliance, huddled together along the horizon. I imagined that some giant broom had swept the stars away from the moon and had piled them in a heap like so much dust in a corner of the sky. Only the constellation Orion challenged the brightness of the moon, for he was armed with two stars of first magnitude, and I could easily identify Betelgeuse, the star in Orion's right shoulder as he brandished his club in the sky in belligerent silence. Orion was the only contentious constellation in the otherwise pacific ocean of sky, and I watched his mirror image in the smooth lake, for there was no stirring of the wind whatsoever to cause warping or distortions in that liquid silvered mirror. I relaxed a few moments alone with the moon and enjoyed the gleaming jewels in Orion's belt with the gentle appreciation of a quiet, loving eye.

Off to Orion's left, I could just barely see the soft fuzz of the Pleiades, that cluster of seven stars on the left shoulder of Taurus the Bull. I tried to identify the stars in Taurus, but the sky was too bright and the best I could do was to see El Nath, the jewel embedded in the very tip of the Bull's left horn.

I had been relaxing in the parked car for almost ten minutes, and when I reluctantly started the engine it shattered the stillness like the crash of a broken mirror, the noise sounding unusually loud to me, perhaps because during my quiet interlude, my ears had relaxed too, and had become accustomed to the total silver silence. I left the lake refreshed; a worthwhile way to spend ten minutes, I figured, even if it was two-thirty in the morning and I had missed a lot of sleep.

I was on my way home from a disgusting call and the fresh cleanliness of the lake, with the stars and the moon-drenched sky, had washed away my irritation and annoyance and had served as an emollient to my wounded mood.

I wished Mr. Stemmler would find another veterinarian. I was convinced the man combined all the qualities of the world's worst farmer, and I loathed working for him because he was filth and laziness personified. The drainage trench behind the cattle stalls, which ran the length of the barn, was always filled to overflowing and brimming with rotted manure, which sat sodden in nitrogenous heaps, well soaked in decomposed urine, where it must have marinated, I judged by the smell, for almost a week. The straw which was supposed to serve as bedding was always saturated with urine and apparently never replaced with clean bedding when it became soiled. The strong ammonia fumes from the decomposing urine had made my eyes water and nose run when I first had entered the barn. The cattle were up to their fetlocks in manure and debris, and when I tried to explain to Mr. Stemmler that the filthy condition of the stalls was the cause of the sore feet and numerous hoof infections his animals had all the time, the farmer shrugged it off and blamed it "to hard luck." He couldn't understand why it was always happening to him, and why he was always "on hard times."

I wasted no sympathy on Stemmler, this man of mean attitudes, with his furtive eyes, sunk deep in fat, where I knew a hundred little lies were hiding. I did, however, fully sympathize with any animal that had the great misfortune of either being born to or sold into this man's overseeing.

The cow I had just finished treating had been easily diagnosed and successfully treated. Ordinarily, this type of case proved to be very gratifying to both farmer and veterinarian because the cure was so prompt and dramatic. When I had been called to treat this cow, I found her not only down, but paralyzed, resting on her sternum with her head twisted to one side so that the muzzle was turned into her flank. The eyes were staring and dull, their pupils dilated; the cow's muzzle was dry and her extremities were cold. She had calved about forty-eight hours earlier, and presented a classic picture of a cow with parturient paresis, or milk fever, a metabolic disorder that frequently developed in cows, usually—but not always—within seventy-two hours after the birth of a calf. Because of sudden profuse lactation, there is an acute drop in the blood serum level of calcium. This sudden production of large quantities of milk frequently takes its toll on the mother, and a cow with milk fever will show an onset of symptoms by staggering and weaving from side to side. There follows paralysis, circulatory collapse, depression, and coma ending in death.

I asked Stemmler if he had noticed his cow staggering earlier in the evening or if there had been any spasms as in tetanus. The man's pig eyes opened a bit in recognition; the cow *had* been weaving, as if drunk, he recollected, but he'd paid it no mind. He had no way of knowing about any spasms, for he had left the animal, returning to the barn shortly before midnight only because he noticed that a light had been left on.

"I only noticed the cow was down because she was in the stall right by the light switch. She was twisted so funny in a peculiar position with her neck kinked like that." He pointed to the contorted animal and continued, "I knew for sure sumpin was wrong for she wouldn't get up no matter how hard I kicked her in the ass." He punctuated his sentence with an expectoration which landed splat in a puddle of ripe urine.

You need the kick in the ass, I thought to myself, as I eyed the helpless beast lying comatose in a sea of saturated, stinking bedding, but aloud I said, "An electric prod or even the devil's own pitchfork won't get this cow up. Can't you see that she is *paralyzed* and can't move?"

I decided not to waste any time talking to Stemmler, but to direct my efforts toward returning the serum calcium level to normal without delay, before I had a dead cow on my hands. I injected the calcium solution into the jugular vein, taking care not to inject it too rapidly lest the animal's great heart go into cardiac arrest. The solution dripped from the half-liter bottle through the tubing and into the cow. The dramatic moment in the cure of a case of milk fever was about to occur, and out of the corner of my eye I watched Stemmler's face. I always enjoyed owners' reactions to the behavior of their nearly dead cow after it received a portion of the intravenous electrolytic solution. How many times did I wish I had a concealed camera to record what was about to happen. By this time, the cow had received about 300 cc of the calcium solution. She sighed and tried to straighten her neck. Next she lifted her head and turned it in front of her in a normal position. She soon discovered that she had a tongue and that it had become wet again, so she used it to lick and moisten her dry muzzle. Her ears twitched and flicked away a fly; they had become warm again to my touch. By the time 450 cc had been given, the cow shifted her ponderous body and with a grunt and expending great effort, she gave a mighty lunge and heaved her rear quarters, raising them so that she half stood, propped up on her rear legs while her front end was still on the ground. There she rested a moment, kneeling on her front legs. Another heave brought the cow upright on all four legs and she stood in her stall, alive once again, and twitched her manure-encrusted tail.

Stemmler had been delighted by his cow's performance. "A meerical" is what he claimed it was, and such terms as calcium, magnesium, hypo or hyper this or that meant nothing to him. What infuriated me most was that I was sure the man was not basically stupid, but that he was just too lazy to try to understand, and my only resort in communicating with him was to stress that in spite of the cow's apparent dramatic recovery, the symptoms could recur, and that he simply had to watch over the animal and pay close attention to how she acted. I warned him that if the animal started to weave and stagger, he should call me immediately and not neglect her again, for the next time he might not be so lucky and his cow might die. Amazingly enough, by the time I had packed my equipment and scrubbed my filthy boots with disinfectant, the cow had given a tremendous belch, regurgitated, and resumed chewing her cud—completely unaware of her recent very close brush with death.

As I was about to leave, Stemmler suddenly assumed an obsequious manner and whined, with a wringing of his dirty hands, "How much do I owe you, Doc?"

I absolutely abhorred this man and I thought quickly of a scheme which I hoped would discourage him from calling me ever again for medical help. Without one moment's hesitation, I innocently asked for a fee three times my usual amount. I smile to myself every time I remember how his pig eyes winced, as an animal's eyes do when it is in pain. But Stemmler didn't say anything, and I hoped that after the elation of the "meerical" passed, he would begin to fume about the bill, and that next time he would call someone else.

Leaving the lake behind, I continued my drive back home, looking forward to a hot shower and a good scrub before going to bed. The morning would come all too quickly to usher in another very busy day.

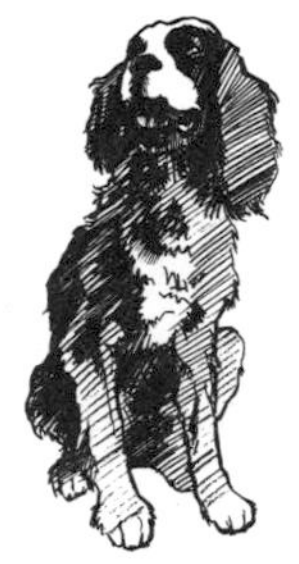

8

I returned the telephone receiver to its cradle. It was a welcome phone call, for it was from Joe, telling me he had just landed, was topping the tanks of his plane, and would be home for dinner shortly. Mame had prepared dinner as far as she could, had set the table and had already gone home. I took a packet of instruments out of the sterilizer and placed a second packet in to cook. As I turned the wheel on the sterilizer door into a locked position, I glanced out the window toward the boarding kennel. The back field was smoldering snow and I could barely discern the black inner-tube swing which Joe had installed several years ago, which was hanging now like a motionless pendulum, patiently waiting for the nudges of springtime and laughing children, which would start it swinging again.

Joe had been away for three weeks on a business trip and I was bursting with exciting news. A possible partner! Free weekends now and then might be just around the corner!

It was a happy reunion and I thought of the German word *gemütlich* as I looked at my family seated at the table. The conversation was lively and continuous and of general interest. We all loved hearing Joe's flying stories; everyone was in high spirits.

About three quarters of the way through dinner, there was a knock on the kitchen door which separated the living quarters of our home from the vestibule that led into the waiting room of the office and hospital. I was about to get up to answer the knock, but Joe suggested, "It's way before hours, honey. Let them wait a bit for once. Finish your dinner."

I was about to comply, when the knocking sounded again, more urgently this time, and Joe started to become annoyed. I shoveled the remaining food from my plate into my mouth under my husband's disapproving stare, and was just getting up when the kitchen door opened.

A young girl of about fourteen entered and started walking through the kitchen toward all of us in the dining room, her face white with fear and shock.

"Please! Oh, please! Is the doctor in?" she asked, tugging nervously at the one heavy braid of hair which draped over her right shoulder and hung down the front of her blue snow jacket.

"My dog has been hit by a car. I'm sure he's going to die!" She did not cry, but her voice was so defenseless and so sad, and there was something about the way her head was bowed when she spoke, with such a complete resignation, that our family unit at the dining table was moved as one person.

I felt a great surge of sympathy for the young girl, and taking her by her hand as I hurried into the kitchen, I asked, "Where is your dog now, dear?"

"About five blocks away on Main Street."

I picked up my bag as I left the office and was surprised to find the girl's parents sitting in their car out in front of the hospital. They hadn't even pulled the car into the driveway and I asked, puzzled, "But where is your dog?" I turned toward the girl. "Is he still on Main Street?"

"Yeah—by the side of the road," answered the father in an annoyed tone.

"But why didn't you bring him with you? I won't be able to do much for him by the side of the road!"

"You see, Pa? I told you," and the girl gave both parents a desperate, imploring glance.

"Button your lip, Miss Prim," quipped her father. "I'll handle this whole thing. . . . Are *you* supposed to be the doctor?" he asked me, as he looked me up and down from head to toe.

"I'm Dr. Logue," I answered, ignoring his remark and his glance. "From what your daughter says, the dog sounds as if it's seriously hurt. Perhaps we'd better not waste any more time."

"Well, O.K.," and he slapped the steering wheel and turned the key in the ignition.

I asked the girl her name, found out it was Honilee, and remarked, "What a pretty name! I've not heard it before. Is it German?" But there was no answer, and next I asked her when the accident had happened. To my dismay, Honilee said that the dog had been hit a good fifteen minutes ago.

"Whatever took you so long to get to the hospital and why didn't you bring your dog along?" I asked again of the father.

"Now look, *missis!"* The man turned his head and frowned back at me, in the rear seat. "Now look here, *missis*"—emphasizing the "missis"—"things are going to be done *my* way! If you *must* know," he continued, his eyes on the road once again, but I could see by means of the streetlights that he kept darting mean looks at me through his rear-vision mirror as he continued talking. "If you *must* know, I didn't want to move the dog. I figured it might hurt him." He added this last bit in a sanctimonious tone that in no way fit his character. "*You* can move him—you're supposed to be a doctor!"

The mirror reflected those eyes again and suddenly I was reminded of Mr. Stemmler and I salivated with dislike.

I could see exactly where the accident had happened by the telltale bloodstains on the newly fallen snow. Already the stain had been mashed into a maroon-colored slush from the continuous traffic which streamed by.

The dog was lying on the side of the road, surrounded by a group of three people—two neighbors, man and wife, and the man who had hit the dog. They were talking to each other in quiet tones.

"Here they are now," I heard one of the men say.

"O.K., everybody, git back! Well, *missis?"* Honilee's father dared, rather than asked the question of me.

Someone had wrapped the dog in a rather expensive-looking woolen blanket, and when I folded back the flap that was covering the dog I saw that the animal's abdominal wall had been ruptured and that the poor creature was almost completely eviscerated, for loops of intestine were lying in ropy coils on the wool. I quickly opened a flask of saline solution and poured it over the viscera to moisten them and wash off gross debris, and then rapidly stuffed the intestines back inside the dog, taping the abdominal wall together in hopes of keeping the guts inside until we reached the hospital. I snapped my bag shut, rolled the dog on its back, and making a sling of the blanket, I grabbed the dog's hind legs along with the blanket and said, "Now, someone, quickly! Take hold of his front legs and the blanket, and let's carry him, blanket and all, to the trunk of the car. Honilee, you support the dog's head, and, ma'am," I asked of the girl's mother, "will you please carry my bag?"

One of the men, the next-door neighbor, helped me and together the three of us started toward the car in quick, short steps, for the dog was large and very heavy. Honilee's father hadn't budged, but remained standing, legs apart and hands on his hips.

"Hurry! Open the trunk quickly. There's really no time to lose!" I knew the dog was dying because of his blanched color and the complete flaccidity of the viscera when I had replaced the intestines in their cavity. The dog's eyes were glassy and I knew that any moment now he would lose consciousness.

"Now just a minute, *missis!* You ain't putting that dog in *my* car!" boomed the owner.

"Put the poor dog down again—gently." I gave a sigh of exasperation, shaking my head. The man who had helped me carry the dog started shouting and reprimanding Honilee's father over my head. From all that he said, I learned that it had been he, the neighbor, who couldn't stand the sight of the intestines lying in the road and, with the help of his wife, had somehow managed to get the dog on one of their blankets and carry him to the side of the road. Evidently, an argument had ensued between the dog owner and the man who had run over the dog. It was obvious to me by now that injury to the dog by moving him had nothing to do with the fact that he had not been brought to the hospital. The owner simply did not want to get his car messed up. However, the main reason the dog was not moved—and this for some reason was more exacerbating than anything else—was that Honilee's father, motivated solely by blind vindictiveness and spite, wanted to cause the driver of the offending car as much inconvenience as possible and had insisted that the man who ran over the dog drive it in *his* car. The driver had refused to do so, stating that it was not his dog, and inasmuch as the animal had not been on a leash, he was in no way responsible. He had made the required phone call to the police and reported the accident. As far as he was concerned, he had done all that he was legally required to do.

And so a quarter of an hour or more had been spent in vicious arguing, each stubbornly refusing the other's requests, until Honilee's father, still not giving in, compromised by driving his wife and daughter to the veterinary hospital, with the intent of passing the whole situation on to the veterinarian.

If I could, which I couldn't, I would have turned on my heel and walked away from them all. But I simply couldn't leave the dog just lying there with its head at Honilee's feet. I glanced up at Honilee—poor Honilee—who was staring straight ahead with her head sagging slightly and tilted to one side. It was painfully plain that this entire horrible situation—both the sight of her neglected ruptured dog and the beastly behavior of her father—were beginning to take their toll on the poor child.

"Will you please drive me to my office?" I asked the neighbor. "I'll bring my car and we can use that—if it's not too late by that time."

"Walter? Take the dog in our car—*please?"* The neighbor's wife blew her nose in her hanky.

"Hell, Doc, I suppose we might as well use our car!" Walter snorted. "This whole thing is making me sick." And speaking over my head again, he continued, "You know, you make me feel sick—real sick? I think you're a disgusting son of a bitch!" Walter shot this to his neighbor and then clamped his cigar stub between his teeth.

"Now looka here, you! Watch that mouth of yours!"

Gentle Jeannie, good as gold, who usually did as she was told, and who had an unusually long fuse, really had had it. My hormones poured forth and filled me with a violent urge to protect Honilee. The mama tiger was aroused and had been spurred into action.

"Enough! Enough, already!" I shouted, and I vaguely remember waving my arms as if I were trying to stop traffic. "Everybody shut up and let's get the dog into the car."

"Just who do you think you are?" started the father again, but that was as much as he got to say, for wanting no more arguments or altercations, I picked up my heavy bag. Swinging myself around in a complete circle to gain momentum, my hair flying, I smashed him in his beer belly with the bag, expelling the hot air from him with considerable propulsion.

"I told you to shut up, didn't I?"

Next, I started on the man who hit the dog. "And you! You

who are so careful to observe your damn legal responsibilities! What about your moral responsibilities? Do you feel anyone has the right to hurt someone so? Look at that girl!" And I pointed to Honilee, who was still standing in the same position. "Either clear out of here, or stop arguing and give me a hand."

His mouth opened twice as if he was going to say something, but no sound came.

Having cleared the air, I went back to the dog, and with Walter's help carried the dog to his car while Walter's wife opened the trunk.

What a way to spend an evening! I thought as I carried the heavy load. How do I get involved in these things, anyway?

Honilee silently supported the dog's head and then stood listlessly by the trunk as her dog's body was laid inside. I saw her eyes flinch slightly as the trunk lid was slammed shut, but other than that, she remained staring blankly, pale and expressionless.

"Would you like to ride in the car with us, Honilee?" I asked, and when she made no reply, I gently took her by the arm. Unresisting, Honilee allowed herself to be led to the car and helped into the back seat, where she sat mute and staring. I looked into her unblinking eyes and saw every misery from the beginning of time puddled in the wide, deep pools of her dilated pupils. I softly stroked a truant strand of hair from the girl's forehead. Her skin was cold and damp. I held her hand and patted it, at a loss for any encouraging words to say to this girl, still a child really, and I put down the awful feeling that before the night was over, I would be more worried about the girl than her dog

The waiting room was full by the time the three cars pulled into the parking area. For some incomprehensible reason, after all the arguing and holding back, both Honilee's father and mother, in their car, and the man who had run over the dog, had followed Walter, his wife, Honilee and myself to the hospital. Walter's wife ran to open the door of the waiting room as Walter and I carried the sagging load in the blanket into the office.

"We'll take him right on into the surgery and put him on the table," I directed as we passed by the concerned and sympathetic faces of clients who were waiting for me with their pets. One man handed his dog to the person next to him and without a word jumped up to lend a hand with the heavy burden.

Once the dog was on the operating table, I swiftly opened the blanket and started shaving the right arm of the dog, hoping that the vein wasn't so collapsed from shock that I would be unable to insert a hypodermic needle.

"I'll be glad to help, if you want me to, Doctor," Walter's wife volunteered. "I'm a registered nurse."

"Why, thank you very much. That would be a great help. I have to get an IV going. Will you help me hold off a vein?"

"Glad to. My name is Betty, by the way." She smiled, took off her coat and pushed the sleeves of her sweater up to just below her elbows. "All right," she said briskly. "Just tell me what to do."

Amazingly enough, there had been no massive hemorrhage, so I knew that the spleen must be intact. Not needing fresh blood with live platelets to aid in the clotting mechanism, we didn't have to spend precious time with a donor dog. We used stored blood serum as a blood expander to elevate the pressure.

I left Betty for a moment and almost immediately returned with a flask of serum which I had taken from my small blood bank. I attached a receiver set of intravenous tubing to the flask, tied a length of gauze bandage to its handle and then tied the flask upside down to the operating room light overhead. I showed the nurse how one holds off a vein in a dog and then tried several times, unsuccessfully, to insert the needle into the collapsed vessel. What a pity! The vein was absolutely flat! I tried another leg.

So we two women, heads bent close and intent on our work, tried again, and all the while we could hear angry voices arguing about who was going to pay the bill for the dog's care.

"Oh, what a miserable man! What a poor excuse for a human being!" Betty exclaimed. "I sure wish we weren't next-door neighbors."

"Is he always this way?" I asked, as I moved to the third leg, the left rear this time. I was still trying to pick up a vein.

"Pretty much so," replied the nurse. "He can pick on the slightest thing and massage it into the biggest argument. He goes into a rage if anyone parks a car by the curb in front of his house. He'll quibble and argue about a quarter-inch deviation in property line. If anyone else's dog or cat comes onto his property, he'll throw something at it, and he doesn't usually miss. He even used a pitchfork once! He's the most vindictive, intolerant bigot I've ever met. He doesn't become red with anger—he becomes white with rage!"

"He sounds sick to me," I murmured, and then, "Ah—here we go," as I saw blood enter the syringe, telling me the needle was in the vein. "Finally!" I disconnected the syringe very carefully from the needle so as not to dislodge it from the vessel, then inserted the adapter end of the IV tubing into the hub of the needle, taking care to expel each little gemlike bubble of air from the tubing first. I secured the needle and the tubing to the dog's leg with strips of adhesive tape and then tied the leg with a length of gauze bandage to a cleat under a corner of the operating table—there was one at each corner. Securing this leg in the proper position, I balanced the dog on its back and tied each of the three remaining legs to a cleat so that the dog's limbs were outstretched.

"Now we can get to the business at hand," I said.

"How fast do you want the serum to drip into the dog, Dr. Logue?" asked the nurse as she started to regulate the pinch valve on the IV tubing by unscrewing it a little. "It seems to be going a bit slowly to me."

"Let it flow at the same rate as you would for a human." I was busy inspecting and cleaning the viscera. I worked as quickly as possible, for I knew I was working against time. The dog was in such a state of shock that it was in another world. It was not unconscious, but it heard and saw nothing. No anesthesia was needed, for the dog was beyond pain. Breathing was dangerously slow and shallow, the corneal reflex was almost nil. "But the dog is still alive," I kept telling myself as I thoroughly checked the entire length of intestine to make sure a resection was not necessary.

It was a situation in which there was everything to gain and nothing to lose, and the fact that the dog still had some slim chance to survive, and the thought of what that survival would mean to Honilee, made me more determined than ever to keep the dog from dying.

"Here's some trouble right here," I said to Betty as I pointed to several torn and severed jejunal arteries. "The bleeding seems to have stopped, but I'm going to tie them off, anyway. They could start bleeding again, especially if and when the blood pressure comes back up."

I started ligating the blood vessels and was pleasantly surprised to find what a help it was having someone hand me the very instrument I needed just as I was about to reach for it myself and pick it up from the instrument tray.

"Why, Betty, I swear you'll spoil me rotten. I never knew what a tremendous help it could be to have a surgical assistant! We veterinarians have to be sort of a one-man band, you know. We're our own prep nurses, anesthesiologists, surgeons, postop orderlies and night nurses all rolled into one. We even have to count our own surgical sponges as we pack them into the abdominal cavity, to be sure we remove the exact number we put in." I looked up at Betty and smiled my appreciation.

"I don't see how you can do all this by yourself," said Betty in disbelief. "I'd be swamped—and I know a number of M.D. surgeons who'd be swamped too. They simply couldn't function under such working conditions. Don't you ever fear you'll become so involved in the surgery that you'll forget to check your patient's breathing, color or IV flow? How much can a person concentrate on at one time?"

I told her that I was always terrified that I'd forget something. It is very easy to become so involved in an intricate bit of surgery that one could indeed forget to check, and there are times in certain surgical procedures when I really should have no distractions at all.

"I have to work with what I've got. It's a question of basic economics. Nowadays pet owners simply can't afford to pay additional fees for an anesthesia man or an OR nurse. They need their money for their children's doctor and dentist bills, for food, clothing, and you know what all."

I asked Betty to check for a femoral pulse, and she said she felt it; it was no prize, but at least it was a pulse. The breathing seemed a little better too.

Maybe he'd make it after all! Oh, how I hoped so—not just because of the medical challenge this type of job presented, but because I would feel so rewarded if I could save this dog for Honilee.

I examined the dog's bladder. Luckily, he had urinated before the accident, for if he had had a full bladder when he was hit by the car, the bladder most probably would have ruptured upon impact and he would have died from shock. There was a slight bruising of the left kidney, but the spleen and liver were intact and he needed no bowel resection, so I really believed that the dog's greatest hurdle was getting out of shock. The fluids were going in nicely and he was in a warm room now.

"We shall just have to wait and see," I said. "Hot intestines slapped onto icy snow would throw any creature into shock!"

We were finished, and suddenly we were both aware of the quiet that prevailed in the waiting room.

"Wonder what happened out there?" Betty jerked her thumb toward the office.

"We'll soon see," I answered. I started preparing a kennel in the recovery room, placing a heating pad on the kennel floor. Next, I took one of my supply of surplus army blankets from a cupboard and draped it over the open kennel door.

"I'll go get my husband to help us carry the dog off the table. If you could carry along the IV set as we move him, I'd appreciate it, Betty."

The waiting room was deserted and I entered the kitchen, seeking Joe. I found him in the living room watching TV, but he was not alone, for Walter and John Hansen were with him. John was sitting in the rocker sucking on his pipe, a new beagle puppy curled in his lap sound asleep. Joe and Walter, both cigar smokers, were puffing away slowly, and all three men were relaxing over cold beers while they listened to the news and excerpts from the President's State of the Union message.

"Hi, John. I didn't know you were here." I nodded to Walter, and then, turning to Joe, I asked him for his help.

As we were walking back toward the surgery, Joe flicked his cigar ash into a handy ashtray and asked, "What in hell happened out here tonight? Jesus H. Christ! It was like a Chinese fire drill! I couldn't get one goddamned thing done on my book, there was such bedlam!"

Damn! I thought to myself with a pang of guilt, for I remembered how Joe had counted on getting so much done this evening on a chapter he was writing for a technical book. He was trying to make up for the three-week interruption his business trip had caused.

"The fighting got so bad I had to come into the waiting

room to see what was going on. It was terrible! A complete waste of time to try to reason with either of those men. The tubby guy was especially obnoxious and I knew that their argument could come to blows. I finally lost patience with them and showed them the door. I felt like a bouncer at some barroom brawl—and in my own home! Christ!"

"Oh, no, Joe! Was it really that bad?"

"You've no idea, Jeanne. For two cents I'd have hauled off and punched that one idiot, but laws being the way they are, I figured I'd end up being the one arrested!"

"Oh, for shame, Joe! You mean you actually thought of striking a blow? You really felt like *hitting* him?" I tucked my tongue in my cheek and glanced at Joe out of the corner of my eye as we passed through the unlit office on our way to the surgery.

The three of us got the large, limp dog safely into the kennel and I covered him with a blanket, tucking him in as gently as I would a child. His foot pads were cold and I gave a worried sigh as I straightened myself up and locked the kennel door. As I went to label the kennel and leave instructions for John, who would arrive in the morning, I suddenly thought of Debbie, his wife. She should have been somewhere on the scene this past evening as receptionist, and now I realized that I hadn't seen her anywhere all during the excitement.

"Say, Joe, did you see Debbie at all tonight?"

"No—she never came."

"Why not? What reason did she give when she phoned?"

"None. In fact, she never phoned," said Joe. "I wouldn't put up with her if I were you."

"Well, now that's it! You're absolutely right! Of all the nights not to show up! I'm firing her in the morning. I've had it with that Debbie." Then I directed my comments to Betty. "Gee, I don't know what name to put on this kennel. I never got the dog owner's name." She told me that the owner's name was Wallace Kidney, and the dog's name was Blackie.

"Hmph," I snorted as I printed KIDNEY on the name tag. "The big bum is shaped just like his name." Betty had to laugh.

Joe explained that John Hansen had entered the office shortly before the two men were evicted, so he witnessed some of the excitement. John and Inga had given their son a new hunting dog for Christmas and John had brought the pup to the office for a distemper shot.

"Ask John to bring the pup in here, will you, Joe? I'll be in with all of you in a minute and I'll fix us all a snack."

I laid several thicknesses of newspaper on the floor, and when John entered the office with the puppy, which was still sound asleep, I took it from him and awakened it gently. I placed it on the newspaper, where it stretched and yawned sleepily. Then it squatted and urinated.

"Housebreaking or paper training a puppy would be so much easier if people would always place the puppy on the paper immediately after it awakens or right after eating. They're just like babies, really. They always wet the diaper after they awaken or right after a bottle!"

The unexpected guests left shortly before midnight, Walter claiming that it was a pleasure to have met us both and that he hadn't had such an eventful evening since the Battle of the Bulge.

Joe and I thanked them for their help and kindness with regard to the Kidneys' dog and Joe turned out the parking lot lights as the cars pulled out of the driveway.

I checked Honilee's Blackie again, turned the heating pad to a low setting, waited a few more minutes until all the fluid finished flowing through the IV tubing and then removed the needle from the dog's vein. I returned to the kitchen and cleaned away the dinner dishes, pots and pans, and then went upstairs to check the children, perhaps to replace a dangling arm or leg in a bed and tuck the blankets around them more securely. I was surprised to find Marilyn awake, and from the disheveled condition of her bed sheets, I knew the child had been restless.

"How come my sunshine girl is not off in dreamland someplace?" I asked, giving her a kiss.

"I just couldn't sleep somehow, Mommy. Are you all right?"

"Of course, Marilyn. I'm fine. Why do you ask?"

"But what was all that yelling and fighting about, Mommy? I could hear them all the way from here!"

I asked her if she remembered the girl who came into our kitchen at dinnertime, and Marilyn said yes.

"Well, that girl's father, I'm sad to say, didn't turn out to be a very nice person. Your daddy made them stop fighting and sent them away. Do you want to get out of bed so that I can smooth your sheets and plump your pillow? Look at it! Like a mashed lumpy marshmallow!"

Marilyn giggled and trotted off to the toilet while I repaired her bed. I tucked her in and as I bent over to kiss her good night, she wrapped her arms about my neck and laughed. "You're locked! You're locked. You can't get away."

And so there was a brief pretended struggle and finally I freed myself. We were both laughing softly in low tones, and the play relaxed and reassured the child.

"Good night now, honey. See you in the morning."

"But what if I can't get to sleep?"

"I'll tell you what to do. It will help you fall asleep. Now shut your eyes"—and Marilyn closed her lids—"and imagine a nice, smooth, round, dark stone lying on the ground. Do you see the stone in your mind?"

"Mm," came the ruffled response.

"Next, imagine snowflakes which are falling from the sky." My voice was murmuring softly now in a singsong, lullaby voice.

"Try counting the snowflakes and keep watching the stone.

Don't take your eyes off the stone, for its dark, round shape will soon grow smaller . . . and smaller . . . as the snow . . . begins to . . . cover it. The stone will get smaller . . . and smaller . . . as the snow continues to fall . . . and silently . . . pretty soon . . . the stone will be hidden, completely covered with snow. There will be nothing but whiteness . . . and you . . . will be asleep." And I tiptoed out of her room.

Showers usually refresh me, but as I finished and started drying myself, I realized that I felt just as tired now as before the shower. Something was bothering me; it was my conscience. I could not relax, and when I canvassed my system to try to understand why I felt ill at ease with myself, I thought of Wallace Kidney and immediately I knew I was going to repent in sore leisure that which I had done quickly in a moment of anger.

I shouldn't have hit him, I thought, as I dried between my toes.

I walked remorsefully across the bedroom, trailing my towel behind me. I sat wearily on the edge of the bed, letting my legs dangle outstretched in front of me with my ankles bent, so that the soles of my feet were staring at each other and the outer edge of each foot rested carelessly on the floor.

Joe glanced at me from his side of the bed, where he was reading while waiting up for me. He saw my head bowed and my chin almost on my chest. He saw my drooped shoulders and the round curve of my spine. He thought I looked unusually tired and somehow penitent and sad, so he put his book aside and asked as he kneaded the small of my back, "What's the matter, Jeanne?"

"Aw, I dunno. . . . Would you dry my back, huh?"

"Well, something is bothering you—I can tell," and Joe rubbed my back soothingly with the towel, not saying another word.

I gave a sigh and confessed that I had done something disgraceful that evening, utterly and unforgivably disgraceful. "I shall never get over it!" I confided.

"Now what could you have done that would be disgraceful?" he asked, as he slid over so that he was sitting next to me on the edge of the bed. He put his arm about me. "Tell me all about it." He brushed back my hair, tenderly kissed my ear lobe, and raising my chin, he also kissed the tip of my nose.

"Well," I sighed, "I hit Mr. Kidney. I *hit* him!" And I turned to Joe with an imploring look. "I belted him right in his midriff!" I looked down at the floor again, more dejected than ever.

Joe maintained a solemn face as he studied me. He kissed me again tenderly and encouraged, "Tell me all about this. I can't believe what you say! Did you actually hit him with your hand?"

"No—I belted him with my bag! With my *bag!* Oh, it's just so awful—and so unprofessional. I'm ashamed to think of it. I don't want to even talk about it!"

"You'll feel better if you do, though." And he pecked me again, this time on my shoulder, murmuring, "Tell me."

"Well," I began lamely, scratching my left heel with the big toe of my right foot, "it was this way." And I recounted the whole thing. "He was just so horrible to Honilee," I explained in conclusion. "I couldn't bear seeing her stand there so dumfounded by hurt. She was so helpless and defenseless. So when I told her father to be quiet and—"

"Quiet?" Joe asked.

"Well, actually, I told him to shut up—but anyway, he wouldn't, so I blew my cool and belted him with my bag."

"Well, now," pontificated Joe, rolling his eyes and raising his brows in a manner befitting a judge. "This sounds as though it might be more serious than I thought." He rubbed his jaw reflectively. "That bag is very heavy. Show me exactly how you hit him, in case it comes to court."

"Court?" I exclaimed in horrified dismay.

"Yes! Court! We have laws. You can't just go around hitting people. Mr. Kidney may press a charge of assault and battery. Show me, in case it comes to court, exactly how it happened."

"Gee, I didn't mean to hurt him. I just wanted to shut him up so we could get Honilee's dog to the hospital. I just got so mad at him, that's all." And I got up, bathed in the lamplight, and using my towel to represent my medical bag, I began to demonstrate.

"You hit Kidney in the stomach in a blind rage? Maybe we can get you a suspended sentence due to temporary insanity. . . ."

But in doing my whirling demonstration, I was just a little bit too fast for Joe. Spinning around just before he removed the grin from his face, I saw a devilish glint of amusement in his eyes.

"Why you! Why you!" and I flew at Joe now as I had at Wallace Kidney earlier in the evening.

"I'll demonstrate to you, all right!" *Snap* and *Whap!* went the damp towel as I chased him around our bedroom. "Oh, you are really something! How could you make fun of me so? How could you enjoy my misery and make light of my baring my soul to you like that?"

Joe let out a whoop of laughter.

"That's not all you were baring to me," and he spanked the skin of my buttock as he collapsed laughing on the bed. He said that he had heard of indignant ladies hitting people with their pocketbooks, but never before with their doctor bags.

"You're usually so calm and placid, Jeanne. In fact, I'll confess, sometimes it is almost to the point of being boring—you're always so goddamn steady all the time. I still find it hard to believe you really hauled off and hit anybody—but I must say it's a refreshing change. I admire you for it. That son of a bitch deserved it, so don't waste any time feeling guilty about what you did to him. Walter told me about the whole thing while you were busy in surgery. It made his day! He said he's even willing to pay part of the bill, he was so gratified by what you did. He said he'd get his money's worth of satisfaction from having seen someone finally stand up to Kidney."

I told Joe he was a first-class stinker for making me confess what he'd known already, then I set the alarm for three in the morning so I could check on Blackie. I snapped off the lamp and settled down in bed, adjusting our blankets. Joe had just about fallen asleep when I whispered in the darkness, "You know what?"

"Now what?"

"Remember you said I shouldn't worry about what I did to Wallace Kidney? Well, I'm not concerned about what I did to Mr. Kidney as much as what I did to myself. I'll never quite forget my hitting him—never."

Joe said I was silly and that I should go to sleep, but sleep did not come.

I tried following the advice I had given Marilyn a while before, and found that it was a good suggestion.

By the time my stone was covered with snow, I was asleep.

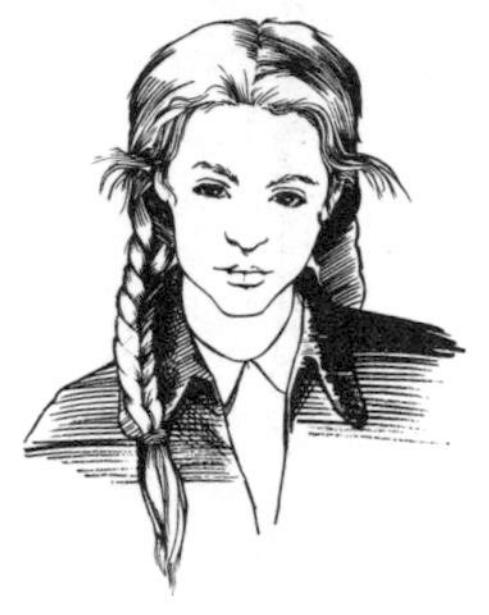

9

The alarm clock and telephone rang simultaneously at six-thirty the following morning. I remembered resetting the alarm when I had returned to bed after checking Blackie Kidney at three, but it took me a few groggy seconds to figure out why the ringing persisted after I turned off the alarm. . . . The phone!

"Good morning. Dr. Logue speaking."

"Missis? This is Kidney. Where's Honilee?"

"Why, I've no idea!"

"Well, she's not at home and the last I saw of her, she was at your place, so I hold *you* responsible!" bellowed Mr. Kidney.

Joe was whispering, "What's the matter. What's up?"

After listening to a spate of self-justifications from Mr. Kidney, I told him I'd let him know if I contacted Honilee and asked him to tell the girl, as soon as she got home, that Blackie was holding his own. I hung up and said to Joe, "I wonder what makes that man tick. I swear he sounded more annoyed than concerned. Honilee is missing."

At the breakfast table, I told Joe, the children, and Mame, who had come from the kitchen to join us for a cup of coffee, the entire story.

"The next-door neighbors and Honilee's parents were all trying to remember when each saw her last. The last *I* remember seeing her was when we were removing Blackie from the car. Betty ran to open the waiting room door, and from that time on I got so involved with the dog—and there was so much commotion and all—well, poor Honilee just seemed to melt into nowhere."

I told them that when Mr. Kidney had finally arrived home, his wife was already in bed. He assumed that she had walked home with Honilee and that the girl was in her room, asleep. Mrs. Kidney, on the other hand, thinking Honilee would wait and return with her father, had walked home alone. It wasn't until the morning, when Mrs. Kidney went to call Honilee for school, that she found her bed hadn't been slept in.

"But didn't she get up to tuck Honilee in when she thought she finally came home with her father?" asked Raymond in disbelief. "You'd think she'd try to comfort the kid about her dog, or something. You mean she just stayed in bed and didn't *do* anything?"

"You mean to say there are ladies in this world who don't tuck?" asked Marilyn incredulously. "Well, now! I think ladies who don't tuck are worse than ladies who spank!"

"That poor child, Dr. Logue!" exclaimed Mame. "Out all night in this freezing weather!"

This last statement was too much for Marilyn to bear. She left the table with a hurried "Excuse me" and returned clutching one of her spayed dolls, which she held tenderly, rocking it in empathy for Honilee.

"You know what I'd do if I were in Honilee's shoes?" asked Raymond. "I'd stay with my dog—that's what."

"I've already thought of that, Ray. But I'm afraid she didn't. She was nowhere around when I checked on Blackie at three this morning."

"Yeah, but—well, suppose she didn't want to be found—didn't want to be sent back home? She'd hide if she heard a noise of someone coming, wouldn't she? If I were her," Raymond reasoned aloud, "I'd hide in a place where no one would think of looking—for a human. I'd hide in that kennel in the corner as you enter the recovery room. When anyone enters they have to open the door, so the kennel is hidden behind it. That would be the place I'd hide—yessiree!"

"Damn it, Ray, you might not have such a bad idea at all! Good thinking," complimented his father.

"Let's all search for the poor child!" said Mame.

"Honilee might be around, but I don't see how she could have prowled through the kennel room at night without setting all the dogs to barking. They barked when I walked through to check on Blackie. I'm alive to that sound and I know I would have heard any barking or unusual commotion all the way from the bedroom. I don't think she's here," I concluded.

"I think it's worth a try, Jeanne," asserted Joe. "I'll check the boarding kennel out back. It's heated, and with all the straw bedding in there, she could easily keep from freezing."

"I'll check the recovery room," said Raymond, and he was off.

"Mame, do you want to check in the skin ward? Check that bathtub too! She could be curled up in that. Marilyn and I will check the main kennel room. Let's all meet back in the office when we're through looking."

And the manhunt was on.

One by one we appeared in the office. First Mame, then Marilyn and I, and next Joe, stamping his feet as he entered the vestibule to get rid of the snow on his boots.

"She's not out back," he reported as he entered the office. "What can be keeping Ray? His is the smallest room of all."

Almost immediately we heard Raymond's voice. He was talking in quiet, encouraging tones and for a moment I thought he was talking to one of the animals, as I had often heard both the children do.

"It's going to be all right, honest. Don't be afraid." And Raymond emerged into the office leading Honilee by the hand.

"Oh, Honilee!" all three females breathed in one voice, and we hovered around the girl like mother hens while Ray and his father stood a short distance aside.

"I found her in the very first kennel I went to, Dad, the one behind the door. She was curled way in the corner, sound asleep. She looked scared when I woke her and I spent all this time talking her into coming out. She acts weird to me, Dad. Won't say a word."

"She's had a very bad experience, Ray," Joe explained in low tones, "and from what I've seen of her parents, it doesn't seem as if her home life is any too stable either. So we just have to try and understand."

I gave Ray a big hug and told him that he was a genius, just like his father. Marilyn decided then and there that her brother would surely grow up to become a detective.

"I was just trying to understand," said Raymond modestly, but proud nonetheless. "I tried to put myself in Honilee's shoes and think as I thought she'd think and do what I thought she would do, that's all."

"You're a hero, you are!" Mame said, and she laid a work-worn hand on Ray's shoulder. "Now I'm going to fix that poor girl a good breakfast, that's what I'm going to do, Dr. Logue."

"Oh-oh! I've missed the bus!" announced Marilyn. We all heard the school bus rumble on its way, and I anticipated that this day, begun with such excitement, was going to be a continuation of the bedlam of the night before.

My estimate proved correct. Everything went wrong. As a start, Joe drove both children to school and was late for an important meeting.

Mame couldn't get Honilee to eat a thing. When I encouraged her to eat some breakfast before she was taken home, the girl still did not utter a word, but she looked so terrified when I mentioned her going home that it upset Mame and me no end.

"Let me fix you a tray and we'll take it into the recovery

room, Honilee. You can eat breakfast while you keep an eye on Blackie. Would you like to plan on coming here every day after school, Honilee? You could help me treat Blackie. Your dog will get better faster with you taking care of him." I kept talking as I carried the breakfast tray into the recovery room, hoping to take the girl's mind off the thought of the confrontation with her parents. I wished I could postpone that ordeal indefinitely.

I wheeled in an instrument table from the surgery and parked it in front of Blackie's cage. Placing a clean towel on the table, I set the tray on top and then brought a chair from the waiting room so the child could eat in some degree of comfort.

"Try to eat something, Honilee—at least drink your orange juice or milk. I won't phone home just yet. I have a few emergencies to take care of first, so you have plenty of time to eat something and visit with Blackie." I figured that at best I could justify postponing that distasteful phone call to the girl's parents for no more than twenty more minutes. I hoped that in that time, Honilee could compose herself somewhat. I cared nothing for Mr. Kidney's feelings, but surely, although the girl's mother seemed to be rather a nonentity, she must possess some love and concern, and certainly had the right to know where her daughter was.

"Pshaw, Dr. Logue. From what I've heard of Honilee's parents, I wouldn't force that child to go home if she didn't want to," advised Mame. "Poor child looks scared to death at the very mention of home!"

"I wish I could squirrel her away in some safe, happy place until I could get her to smile and talk again. Maybe she'll start talking to her dog. . . . Perhaps Blackie will wag his tail or whimper a cry of recognition. That might bring her around."

I took a deep breath, picked up the phone and then replaced

it in its cradle without asking the operator for the number.

"Oh, Mame, I simply hate to phone her parents—they just don't seem to care about her. That mother seems to be in another world. Honilee is acting just like her. She's escaping by clamming up and backing off from everything. The father needs a prefrontal lobotomy, as far as I'm concerned. What a pitiful mess they're all in. I really believe that in addition to love, the girl needs psychiatric help. On second thought, I guess the parents need it too."

"You do what you think is best, but I wouldn't phone 'em." Mame was absolute and took a firm stand, her righteous indignation expending itself in an unusual clatter and rattling of dishes.

I cast about in my mind, hoping to find the best solution to Honilee's problem. I decided to check once again on the girl to see if her spirits had improved any.

I returned to the kitchen and walked toward the phone. "No luck," I reported. "No response at all. She hasn't touched her food. She's just sitting there staring at that dog. Damn! I wish he'd give her just one little wag—one lousy little wag! This certainly isn't my type of day." I continued to unburden myself to Mame. "To make matters worse, neither John nor Debbie has arrived for work yet!"

"That means the dogs haven't been let out yet," said Mame, knowing the consequences when the kennel man was late. "I'll let them all out right now, Dr. Logue. And don't you mind me, dear," she said, patting my shoulder in a motherly fashion. "I'm sorry for sounding so critical of your phoning the girl's parents. I know you have to do what you think is right."

The phone call was made, and with a heavy heart I went to tell Honilee that her father would be along shortly to take her home. At first the mother had suggested that I send Honilee home, but this I refused to do. I was shocked at the very idea of having the girl walk all that way alone after the experience of the night before, and I declined to drive her myself, figuring I'd keep Honilee with me as long as possible, until one or the other of her parents came for her. Honilee's mother had finally decided to phone her husband at work and had told me he'd come for her as soon as he could.

I started treating hospitalized animals all by myself, hoping Mr. Kidney would have come and gone before clients started filling the waiting room.

The way the door opened and closed was an announcement in itself, and I went to speak to him.

"Where is she?" Mr. Kidney's voice expressed neither relief nor joy, nor gentleness, nor love, and my heart quailed at its coldness. I mentally cowered, almost losing courage in my conviction that what I was doing was best for Honilee. But if I feared the concept of such human coldness, I did not fear the man himself; and I took a few quick, commanding steps toward him. My mama tiger was up again. I desperately wanted to help and protect Honilee, but all I could do anymore was to say, "Please be patient with her. You must be gentle and kind to her. Do you understand?" I hissed my intensity at him. The man looked at me, a woman. I must have suddenly reminded him of a mean goose hissing, protecting her eggs.

I considered the futility of my efforts. One cannot compel kindness or love as one can command obedience, I concluded in silence, and I left to get Honilee.

"Honilee doesn't seem to hear, Mr. Kidney," I told the father when I returned without the girl. "You really should call a doctor; she's ill. She's just sitting there—"

"I'll doctor her, all right!" and he started toward the recovery room.

"Not a single word!" I hissed.

And there was just that. Not a single word. He strode through the rooms, took Honilee firmly by the arm and marched out, never bothering to close the door behind him.

Oh, his silence was a vituperative thing, and it crept like poisonous gas across the floor and around the chairs. It entwined the drapes and ensnared the lampshades and then adhered to the walls and ceiling, damp and cold. I shivered and suddenly realized that the door was still open, letting in the freezing January air. As I went to shut the door, I caught a glimpse of Mr. Kidney and Honilee, who was still in her blue jacket, for she had worn it all night. That firm grip remained on her arm, but her father let go of her as he opened the car door. And there was a swift blue flash, like a blue jay in flight, as Honilee bolted, and like a frightened bird, flew away.

I was about to follow her, but thought the better of interfering in their lives any further. I had tried my best, and decided to turn my mind to my own business.

I was about to phone John when I heard squealing brakes and a crash.

Mame came running from the main kennel room.

"What was that? It sounded like an accident. So close—like just outside!"

I was already out the door. Mame followed, and together we ran, coatless, to the street in front of the house.

It was a two-car accident; Honilee had been caught in between.

"Oh, Mother of Jesus! It's Honilee!" wailed Mame.

Honilee's father had recourse to just one form of expression. The air was bombarded with such profanity and blasphemy that the snow seemed to start to melt. I helped a hysterical woman out of the car in the left lane.

"He suddenly swerved into my lane right in front of me!" she screamed. "He came out of nowhere!"

I instructed Mame to lead the woman into the office and, after seating her, to phone for an ambulance and the police.

I checked on Honilee immediately, but could do absolutely

nothing for her because the child was pinned under one car. A white, panic-stricken face was behind the wheel. The driver wound down his window.

"She ran right out in front of me! I couldn't help hitting her! I pulled to my left to try to avoid her, and hit a car coming toward me in the opposite lane. I just couldn't avoid hitting the girl." The driver was jabbering now. "I'll back up and free her!" he yelled.

"My God! *No! No!* You'll run over most of her again!" I straightened myself and stood up, looking down the road, shading my eyes with my hand in hopes I'd catch sight of the ambulance, even though I knew it couldn't possibly arrive so soon. I squinted in the glare caused by the sun on the snow.

The driver got out of his strangely familiar car, and to my sick amazement and utter disbelief, I found myself looking into the pale, horrified face of the man who had run over Blackie the night before. I remember that he took just one uncomprehending look at Honilee in her blue jacket, at her father, at both cars, and immediately started retching. He pitched forward and fainted, falling noiselessly into his own vomitus on the snow-covered ground.

A siren was heard and suddenly everyone was there: doctors, police, a tow-truck crew and people—crowds and crowds of curious people.

They started jacking the car up in order to free Honilee, and when this was done she was transferred onto a stretcher. The girl and the man who ran over her were carried into the ambulance, and Honilee's father followed.

As the ambulance door was about to close, I caught sight of Mr. Kidney's face. He was not bending over his daughter, but was staring in hatred at the unconscious driver, and I felt that had this man been awake, Honilee's father would have resumed the whole horrible argument of the night before—only today it would have been over a daughter instead of a dog.

Somehow we got through the day. John and Debbie did not appear at all and no one answered their phone. I finally gave up trying to reach them. Mame helped me with cases I could not treat alone and when the children arrived home from school, Raymond cleaned kennels. Mame fed the dogs and Marilyn the cats. I rescheduled a farm call I had that day and refused any further calls, referring them to the veterinarian in the next town.

The next day was no better. Again John and Debbie did not appear, and in disappointment and despair, I phoned the employment service for both a kennel man and a receptionist. I might expect Debbie to pull a stunt like this, but dependable John? Something must be terribly wrong. I was disillusioned, tired and unhappy as I completed my conversation with the employment agent.

The phone shrilled at me immediately after I hung up.

"Dr. Logue speaking," I answered mechanically.

"This is Betty Schroeder—the nurse who helped you with Blackie, remember?"

"Of course, Betty. Any news of Honilee?" and I heard a sequence of sobs over the phone. When her voice regained composure once again, I learned that Honilee had died the previous evening.

"She had a ruptured spleen. What with the massive internal hemorrhage, shock and, of course, the stress she had been under, she just couldn't cope with it all. I was on duty yesterday and had her as a patient. She regained consciousness just once for a brief moment and—and—" Betty started crying again, but finally got her story told. "She looked up at me with those haunted eyes and asked me a question—one word: 'Blackie?'

That's all she ever said. Oh, Jeanne, I feel ill—just sick about the whole thing."

For the second evening in a row I couldn't eat very much at dinner, and that night in the darkness of our room, during that quiet time before one falls asleep, I asked my husband, "Did I do wrong? Did I do wrong phoning Honilee's parents?"

"No, you did not," answered Joe firmly. "You did the best you could. She would have had to return to her parents sooner or later, no matter what you did yesterday."

"I think so too," and I sighed as I rested my head on his left shoulder and laid my arm across his chest. "I just needed a little moral support, I guess. So enough now of my moping. I was involved in something I didn't ask to be involved in and I did what I thought was best. If what I did was wrong, I did wrong and I cannot undo it. So it is done and I guess I shouldn't heap any more ashes on myself in penitence. I've made everyone around here miserable for the past two days and this mustn't go on. . . . But oh, dear, when I think of the last words I heard that man say to his daughter, I swear it's enough to make me cry."

"What was that, Jeanne?" Joe asked.

"He snarled, 'Button your lip, Miss Prim!' And you know what, Joe? She did just that! I never heard another word out of her. Poor Miss Prim . . . she buttoned her lip forever."

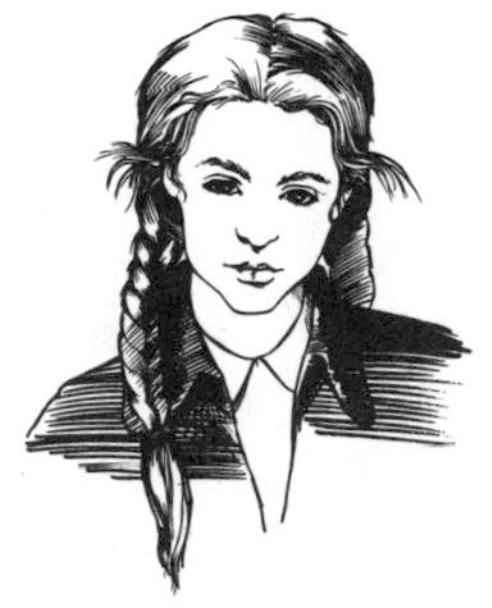

10

When the family was at breakfast the next morning, everyone was surprised to hear dogs barking. I checked and returned to the table.

"John's back! I saw him letting the dogs out of the boarding kennel, as usual. I wonder what reason or excuse he'll give for not coming to work Tuesday or Wednesday."

"Are you going to fire him, Ma?" Raymond asked me.

"We'll see," was all I could say to him. "We'll see."

I was about to ask John where he and his wife had been and reprimand him for not phoning, but I held my tongue when I caught a glimpse of his face. How he had changed! He was no longer the boyish young man I'd seen Monday, but looked old and tired. Creases ran from his nose down along each corner of his mouth, which was clamped shut in a grim, unhappy line, and under his eyes were dark circles which gave them a hurt, hollow look. The rings beneath his eyes were of a grayish-purple color and reminded me of how tissue looks when badly bruised. Indeed, his whole being looked bruised as he went about his chores in a beaten, apathetic manner.

"Now, there's a man with the whole world on his mind," I said to myself, and all thoughts of admonishment were completely gone. Greeting him with as much cheerfulness as I could muster without sounding artificial, I said, "Good morning, John. Good to have you back." I pressed him for neither explanations nor excuses. John answered me with a muffled grunt and disappeared into the main kennel room, to be about his work.

I warned Mame to back off from John and briefly explained how he looked, commenting that it would seem as though he must have had his own peck of trouble these past few days.

A young woman sent by the employment agency came to be interviewed. Her name was Agnes Brown and she was well named, for she had nice brown hair and brown eyes. A big plus was that she raised Kerry blue terriers and was trying to get her own kennel established. Miss Brown did not object to the odd hours and the various services I would require of her, so I hired her on the spot and started training her in our office routine. The morning, for the first time all week, started to pass uneventfully, affording me hope that I could get John straightened out and my practice on an even keel again. The phone rang.

"It's for you, Doctor," said Agnes. "It's a Mrs. Kidney and she wants to speak only to you."

"I'll take it on the other extension, Agnes. I'll show you our filing system later."

"Dr. Logue?" the timid voice asked when I picked up the phone.

"Yes, Mrs. Kidney. Is there anything I can say or do to help? Your neighbor told me the sad news."

"Well, yes, there is." The little mouse sounded less frightened now. "I don't know quite how to explain, but you see—well, I'd like somebody to be at my Honilee's funeral. You seemed kind to her. Do you think—do you suppose you could come? I just can't bear to be alone there with only Mr. Kidney. I—" Her voice cracked and there was silence.

I was appalled at the thought of the two lonely figures at

the grave site and said I would surely attend the funeral. I asked if there was any family member I could contact for her.

"Oh, no . . . no. If you could just come."

"Your next-door neighbor loved Honilee. I'm sure she'd want to attend the funeral too."

"That would be nice. I'd take comfort in that. Somebody should come for my Honilee—but don't let on to Mr. Kidney that I asked you. Just come," Honilee's mother pleaded.

"If any question arises, I'll just say we wanted to come, and that will be the truth." I asked her about the necessary details and then I phoned Betty. I promised to call for her in my car at the appointed hour the following day.

I told Agnes that I would accept no further large-animal calls until the following Monday and that I would not be holding office hours on Friday afternoon because I was going to attend a funeral.

I went into the main kennel room. It was high time John and I started treating the hospitalized animals.

"Almost ready to help me with cases, John?"

He answered me with a grunt which I assumed was meant as an affirmative. Suddenly all my high resolve to mind my own business about his private troubles dissolved as I sensed his utter, entire sadness. "John, what is the matter?" I asked. "We've worked together almost every day now for eight years. I feel we're friends and hope you feel that way too. You can talk to me about whatever your problem is if you want to. Maybe I can help."

"Naw. Thanks anyway, Dr. Logue, but there's nothing you can do." And I was about to say that in that case we had better turn our thoughts to treating cases, but John, after taking a deep breath, continued to talk.

"I see you got a new girl and that's good, 'cause—'cause Debbie's gone. Debbie up and left me—ran away with another man." His voice trembled with emotion and the cruel hurt of his wife's contemptible form of rejection.

"How can you be sure, John? Maybe she—"

"No, ma'am—she left a note." And John, once over the hurdle of hearing his own voice speak the awful news to someone for the first time, was able to talk more easily now. He told me how Debbie had left their house that past Monday evening. He thought she was going to work because she left at her usual time, but she never returned. He had become worried when it grew very late, so he went to phone the office to see what could be keeping her, and discovered her note next to the phone.

"She wants a divorce," he said miserably.

"She must be out of her mind," I sympathized, "to give up a fine person like you. You're a good husband and father, I'm sure— But where is the baby?" I asked in sudden alarm.

"Joy is with me. Debbie deserted us both," he said sadly. "Debbie's mother is minding Joy. Oh, Dr. Logue, I've looked everywhere for her! All Monday night, all day Tuesday and Wednesday. I couldn't sleep at all last night. . . . There's not a trace of her. I just wish she'd come back!"

"If that is what you truly want, then I hope she comes back too. In the meantime, don't slam any doors. If just one of you can keep the door open long enough—no matter what things happen—then you might have a chance of getting back together again. So come now, John, let's pick up the pieces. We've had trouble here ourselves while you've been gone and there's a lot to be done. Bring in the Kidney dog first for treatment, will you, John?"

Blackie was progressing nicely, but I felt a deep sadness because Honilee would never know that in time her dog was going to be all right.

It was snowing again as the group of five adults, plus the gravediggers, stood by Honilee's grave site. The funeral director said a perfunctory prayer as they lowered her coffin, and the snowflakes kissed Honilee goodbye.

For a moment, I thought that Betty and I were the only ones present who were moved by what was happening. Then I saw the wince and slight narrowing of Mrs. Kidney's eyes every time the shovelfuls of earth hit Honilee's coffin. Her eyes reminded me of Honilee's eyes and how they had flinched that moment when the trunk lid was slammed shut on Blackie the previous Monday evening.

By the time we all turned to leave, there was a light frosting of snow on the fresh mound of earth.

Mr. Kidney strode over to the gravediggers, Betty Schroeder walked on ahead toward the car, wiping her eyes, and Mrs. Kidney and I had a brief moment alone together.

"Thank you for coming, Doctor. I know you must find it hard to understand Mr. Kidney's manners, and perhaps even my actions too."

"Yes, I do," I answered quietly. "I find it very hard to understand how any man can be so cold and indifferent to his own daughter! I—"

"But that's just it! You see, Honilee was not his daughter! Oh, I had frantic hopes that the baby would be born late and somehow he would never know, but she was born during our seventh month of marriage—a big, full-term baby—and oh, she was so beautiful!" And the mother's tears finally flowed. "Mr. Kidney never forgave us," she continued after blowing her nose. "He has never let Honilee or me forget what I did. He's been punishing both of us ever since, over all these years."

I swallowed hard, fighting to say the right words.

"Mrs. Kidney, I still find it hard to believe a man could be so cruelly cold to his own daughter—no matter who the father was!"

"Come on, missis," Mr. Kidney said brusquely. "Time to git goin'."

His wife turned, and without another word silently followed him.

I stood still and watched them disappear, and their receding figures dissolved in the swirling snow.

They're both as dead as Honilee, I thought to myself. They are both dead and they're driving to their empty house on Main Street.

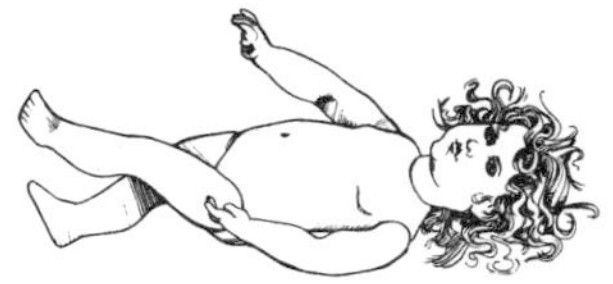

11

Everything was coming back to life. The snows melted, the ground thawed, and the last ice crystals left the soil spongy and porous-looking. It was soft, and yet it looked hard like coarse pumice, and the ground reminded me of lava.

The spring rains fell from acres of well-seeded clouds, and streams and rivers overflowed their banks until the earth became waterlogged. Beneath the ground a mirror image of the activity above was going on. Tree roots collected and drained the area of water just as their sister river-systems were doing on the surface. The water flowed up through the tree trunks and emptied into massive deltas of newly formed leaves, which lost the water by evaporation, and so the billions of leaves, like billowing green clouds, rained invisible raindrops back into the sky.

Springtime! And once again the wonder of it all!

The melting snows helped wash away sad memories of January's tragedy. Blackie Kidney had miraculously recovered and John took him home. Blackie made a fine pet for his little girl.

It was spring recess. Marilyn was on the porch with two girlfriends. They were playing with their dolls, and Marilyn's voice came floating through the window as she chanted in a singsong voice:

"I never saw a purple cow,
I never hope to see one,
But I can tell you right now—
I'd rather see than be one!"

The girls left the porch and gathered on the grass outside the surgery window, where I could see them. Janice, the girl next door, was proudly showing off her doll's new Easter outfit.

"My mother made it for her," she said, turning the doll around to show her off.

Marilyn admired the pretty pink dress with the lace trim and the hand-knit dainty angora sweater and matching bonnet.

Rose's doll was also well dressed, but instead of modeling her doll, Rose modeled herself. Evidently her mother was talented too. Rose preened and pirouetted to flair the full skirt her mother had made for her. It had red and white stripes and the swirling child looked like an animated barber pole. Flushed and smiling, she finally sat down next to Janice, and together they looked expectantly at Marilyn. And what could Marilyn show them that her mother could do? They looked down at her doll. It was stark naked.

"What can your mother do, Marilyn?"

Marilyn was at a loss for words. What *could* her mother do? Her own outfit was store-bought and her doll was naked. The only adornment it had was a red splotch of Merthiolate on its abdomen, marking the site of its most recent spay operation. Her mind raced to find something—*anything*—that her mother had ever done which could approach the cleverness and skill of Rose's and Janice's mothers. Marilyn was losing face fast and beginning to feel very insecure, but then her face flooded with a look of relief. She must have remembered a fragment of conversation she had overheard the day before in the waiting room, which ended with something like: "What? Dr. Logue can do that too?" and then: "Yes! Isn't that absolutely amazing? You'd never think it possible, to look at her."

Confident of her status now, she pulled her skirt neatly over her bare knees and said, "Well, now, can either of your mothers castrate a horse?"

"Why—why, no," admitted Janice in a somewhat deflated voice.

"N-no," from Rose, whose eyes were puzzled and wondering.

"Well," said Marilyn, with a smug smile and confident toss of her head, *"mine can!"*

A few days later, Marilyn, a spayed doll dressed for the occasion, and our German shepherd, Star, were riding along on a call out to the Boldingers' goat farm. Star loved riding in the car and showed it, her mouth partially open in a carefree smile and her huge pink tongue hanging out like a large salami.

Marilyn carried on a continuous monologue, and I'd nod my head and smile from time to time to show I was paying attention. Star would always outdo me in convincing Marilyn that she had the proverbial canine's ear. The dog would nod her head and smile too, but she would also wag her tail.

Mrs. Boldinger supplemented the family income by raising goats and selling the goats' milk and cheese she'd made from it. Parents of children who were allergic to cow's milk sought out Mrs. Boldinger, but many others consumed her products. It was kind of a gourmet fad in the area and Mrs. Boldinger made out very well with her small business. But the thing she liked most about the business, she told me once, was that it reminded her of goatherding in Switzerland when she was a little girl. She had a smooth, round face with merry blue eyes and always wore a triangular kerchief around her head. Every trip I ever made there made me feel as if I were stepping into the pages of the book *Heidi*. Just about everything pertaining to Mrs. Boldinger was clean. Her apron was always clean, as were her pots, her pans, her buckets, her ladles and, of course, the gleaming milk cans. The whole place smacked of lots of soap and water.

There was a case of dystocia which required attention, and after sudsing with disinfectant and rinsing, I inserted my hand and arm into the goat and felt around for the little kid within. I found twins, clinging to one another as if in fear of the momentous journey ahead, which would wash them out into a strange, cold place. After all, in here they were moist and warm and cozy, so why leave?

The Boldingers' two grandchildren were visiting, and together the three children watched the procedure in silent wonder. Because of them I was relieved when I found I could easily disentangle the reluctant twins and deliver them without too much struggle. I wanted this exciting occasion to have a happy ending.

"Oh!" came the awed chorus from all three children as the first baby goat came out. Then came the second one. The two newborn kids squirmed a bit, managed to get on their knees and stand up, quivering and shaky, but seeming to gain moral support from each other as they stood very close together. And then they were grinning at each other as if agreeing, "It wasn't so bad after all, eh? You hungry too? Let's try a bit of this"—and they wobbled to their mother's flank and started smacking away at her udder with noisy gusto.

Without a sound, my Marilyn ran to me and hugged me. She remained just so, holding me tightly, staring at the newborn creatures. I wrapped my arms around her and held her too, and we smiled into each other's eyes.

There was no need for words.

But after a bit, the questions came.

"What? They've been in a sac of water all that time?"

"Yes."

"But why?"

"It's nature's way. It protects the young as they develop and cushions the soft bones so they're not pressed and molded against the hard, firm bones of the mother's body. It prevents the bones from becoming misshapen. The fluid is a water cushion which acts as a bumper and a shock absorber."

"But why the gush when the baby is born?"

"To lubricate the passage and make slipping out easier."

And on and on. They wondered at everything and were shocked at nothing. Everything seemed to have a purpose and each child gained faith in "nature's way."

I loved being with children and still do. I feel very relaxed and comfortable with them. My own simple childish enthusiasm for all these things I do has never slackened. I can let my emotions hang out unabashed with kids around, for I feel with them the magic of childhood—curiosity, great empathy and the art of simple acceptance.

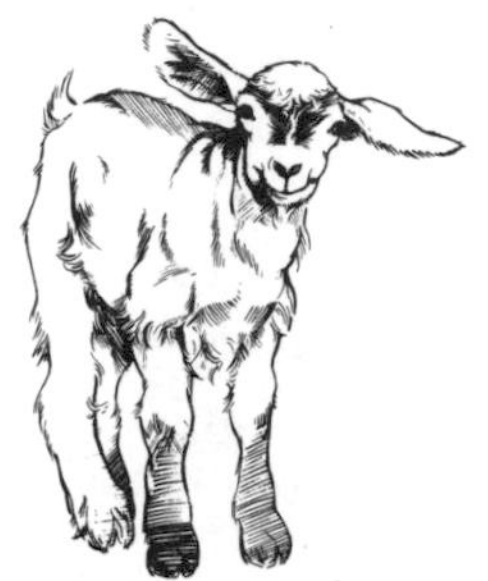

12

Ralph Dorsey was a mild-mannered, friendly soul whose congenial face was usually wreathed in smiles. He customarily laughed words rather than spoke them. Up and down the words would roll, loud then more softly his laughter would peal. He had a gift for making every day a holiday.

Gloria and Charlie Sentell, their two children, Joe, Ray, Marilyn and I were on our way to the Dorseys' one summer Saturday for some swimming and a picnic. Ralph and his wife, Joan, had sold their house in town in order to purchase a very old, very decidedly run-down farmhouse, which came with multitudes of colorful, self-seeded hollyhocks from years past, a barn and lots of land. The big bonus was a broad, clear creek, excellent for swimming. As soon as we arrived at the Dorsey estate, everyone scrambled in for a swim.

Ralph sat in an inflated black inner tube and floated on the water, laughing as he described the big plans they had for their place—how they were going to modernize and redecorate the house, keeping in mind the craftsmanship of the old place, how they were going to repair the old barn and add some dairy cattle to their collection of animals, which already consisted of a number of black Aberdeen Angus beef cattle, some chickens, a rooster and a number of questionably desexed capons (Ralph had purchased a caponizing kit and had removed only one testicle from each bird), two Morgan horses, three bloodhounds, and a miscellaneous assortment of cats, all of which Joan insisted on keeping.

"Take them to Jeanne and have them all spayed, then," Ralph once suggested, "so we don't keep getting more all the time! Pretty soon we'll be overrun with cats!"

And in dribs and drabs they had brought them to my surgery. But always one or two females had been overlooked or mistaken for males when the time came for the mass surgery, and invariably Ralph and Joan would be right back where they started as soon as the next mating season came around.

The next resort had been to gather into several large portable kennels all the cats that hadn't been attended to and ship them off to the hospital at the same time. I spayed or castrated all but one very old tom and their original cat, Mandy, who was now seventeen years old. I hadn't been able to fish out any uterus or ovaries in two of the younger cats, and after probing in vain for about half an hour, I closed the tiny flank incision and in desperation cut a big midline opening down the belly of each cat. With this panoramic view of things, I soon saw that there were no genital organs left in either one and it was then I realized that these two cats must have been two of my previous patients, mistakenly mixed in with the new batch.

Embarrassed, I had been all apologies. "Gee, I'm sorry, Ralph. I couldn't see any scar when I shaved them and I had no way of knowing these two had been done before."

Ralph didn't seem to mind. He had watched me spay a cat once and evidently remembered the shaving and cleaning of the cat's left flank, the emptying of its bladder, and the small slit, a quarter to a half inch in length, that had been made in the skin.

"I remember the one precisely placed stab wound Jeanne

made through the cat's abdominal muscles and peritoneum," he once told a friend. "Nothing else was cut and the incision was enlarged just by stretching the tissues. Next came the spay hook—it looks like an old-fashioned button hook. She inserted it in the cat, moved it around in a certain way, and by golly, when she withdrew it, there was one horn of the uterus caught in the hook. The entire uterus and both left and right ovaries were removed from this one tiny opening."

My use of suture material that in time would be absorbed, and the rapid healing of the flank incision, enabled Ralph to understand why I had no way of knowing just by looking at it, months later, from the outside, whether a cat had been spayed. Actually, Ralph had enjoyed a hearty laugh about this whole incident, and the mere thought of me standing in the surgery, poking around like a mad thing with my spay hook and repeatedly coming up with nothing, wondering where in hell the uterus was and what had gone wrong, caused him to collapse into uncontrollable fits of laughter. For years after, Ralph took great glee in telling this story (which he entitled "The Cats Which Were Spayed Twice") over and over again to anyone who would listen.

Now Ralph was preparing a mess of steaks for dinner, his face wreathed in smiles of honest pride, for the meat was from steers the Dorseys had raised.

"We're serving a dinner off the land tonight," he announced with great satisfaction. "My beef and Joan's vegetables. This is how we all live down on the farm!" and he literally danced with his steaks to the grill.

"Shall I round up the children?" Gloria asked of Joan.

"No, I'll get them, thanks. I know just where they are."

As she was about to go off, there commenced a screeching and a yelling such as none of us had ever heard before. Such terrified, panicky screams they were! We parents were frightened now and even Ralph looked grim as we all tore after

Joan, who was running as fast as she could toward the barn.

The screaming and crying continued, but now peculiar, more horrifying sounds could be heard as we neared the barn. There were strange gurglings and gaggings, and the stertorous, interrupted sounds of labored breathing. There was also a steady but erratic walloping noise and a scuffling, as if some wild animal was thrashing about.

Joan's favorite Morgan mare was lying on the ground just outside the barn door, spewing red froth from her mouth and nostrils. She was on her right side and her legs were flailing in a galloping motion, getting her nowhere.

Joan was crying now, her head pressed between her hands, and wailed, "Angel! Oh, Angel!"

The mare attempted to respond to her name and pathetically tried to determine where Joan's voice was coming from by twisting her head in a weaving motion, up and back. Then the head would smack on the ground, and all the while the animal's terrified eyes, with only the whites showing, rolled around in their sockets and glared at nothing and everything, seeking wildly for Joan's voice. Each time the mare would fling her head there was a pink spray that spumed into the air, which almost immediately dissolved into nothingness, like a cloud of aerosol mist.

All the children were spattered with blood, and they stood screaming at the spectacle, their bare legs dangerously close to the thrashing hoofs. Only Raymond and the Dorseys' oldest boy, Jack, stood transfixed, staring in numb silence down at the struggling mare. Joe quickly moved the children back and Gloria, trying her best to calm them, herded them away.

From the way the horse was suffocating, I knew she must have a collapsed trachea. I felt sick as I noticed a strand of very strong wire stretched tightly across the barn doorway, just high enough to reach the horse's throat, which I saw was cut deeply and bleeding badly. Surely the horse must have come racing toward the barn door, and not seeing the wire, ran right into it.

"Ralph!" I hollered. "Go and cut an eight-inch length from the best section of your garden hose."

"What?"

"Yes. An eight-inch length—and not from any perforated, leaky portions either. Hurry!" And then to Raymond: "Come with me and help me carry stuff from the car."

Joe was already on his way toward the trunk, and together the three of us brought an assortment of ropes and bags over to the mare. I told Charlie to lie down and put all his weight on the horse's neck and head.

"Hold her head down so she can't raise it and thrash it around anymore." I was down on the ground now beside Charlie, and after wiping away the blood in order to see what I was doing, I began infiltrating a local anesthetic into the tissues on either side of the midline of the throat, around the injury, then along and down to about four inches below where the wire had cut.

"What's that you're using?" asked Charlie.

"Two percent procaine."

"But isn't that what they use on us?"

"Sure—it's exactly the same," and I got up and went to the ropes. While the procaine was taking effect, I roped the horse's legs, and with Ralph's and Joe's help, trussed up the poor animal as if it were to be gelded. By good coincidence, I had most of the equipment I needed on hand, for the waiting room had been full when I returned from castrating some horses the day before and I had been too busy to unload the car. I took a knife and made a lengthwise split in four inches of the eight-inch length of garden hose Ralph had brought me. I unwrapped a clean scalpel from a surgical pack, and kneeling next to the mare, I carefully made a three-and-one-half-inch incision directly along the midline of the mare's throat.

What a difference between this mad scene and the first time I did this procedure as a surgical exercise at school! Everything was calm and well organized then. A nice, uninjured cooperative horse was securely restrained and the whole operation, done while the horse stood in a convenient position, was accomplished in quiet comfort. The only inconvenience during my first tracheotomy operation was that my arms were bent and raised a bit during the surgery, so that the blood trickled down my forearms and dripped from my elbows.

Remembering that the median raphe is supposed to be a relatively insensitive tissue, I knew that if I could keep on it, much less anesthetic would be needed. But I soon found that it was a lot easier to stay on the midline when a horse was standing; indeed, my position on the ground was a very awkward one in which to work. I was convinced that I'd end up with a case of housemaid's knee.

I exposed the trachea by blunt dissection and then cut a little oval window in it involving two consecutive cartilaginous rings, neither of which had been cut completely through. Already the mare's breathing was easier and less labored as she gratefully sucked in great tidal volumes of air and then blew them out again through her newly made blowhole.

Charlie, still holding down the horse's head, had shut his eyes the minute he saw the scalpel start the skin incision. He averted his head and opened his eyes now and found himself staring into the large brown eye of the mare. Her eyes were no longer lolling around in her head, and all Charlie could see was the soft limpid brown of the iris and the absolute blackness of the dilated pupil staring at him. The mare held him with her velvet eye and Charlie started to talk to her softly, and his voice had a soothing effect.

I inserted the unsplit end of the garden hose into the mare's windpipe, and bending each of the exposed split ends, one upward and one down, I anchored the hose in place by sewing each end to the skin, thus maintaining an open air passage.

It was a crude procedure, perhaps, but effective, for I had no tracheotomy tube with me and so had to improvise, doing the best I could with what was on hand.

After repairing the collapsed portion of the trachea and removing one loose spicule of cartilage, I trimmed the ragged edges of the wound and sutured the skin together.

"There you are, Angel! You're all neat and tidy and you can breathe again." And then to the rest, "O.K., let's get her up."

One by one we undid the ropes, Charlie holding down her head till the very last.

"All right now, Charlie, let her go and let's everyone stand back and see if she wants to get up."

We watched the horse carefully and saw that she seemed to have control of her senses now as she started to rise, apprehensively at first, but in a collected manner. As we continued to observe, I was moved by love for the beast as I saw her shake herself and try to make the best of things.

I suggested to Jack that he get a rub rag from the barn. The horse was wringing wet with sweat and had to be dried.

"No, I'll do it." Joan was composed now and wanted to busy herself by doing something.

"No, Mom! I want to do it. I'll help her. I'll rub and walk her till she's dry, even if it takes me all night."

"No, I will, Jack. It's my horse."

"Mom? I will! I just gotta. *Please?*"

Raymond appeared surprised that his friend, such a big boy, was actually on the verge of tears.

"Why all of a sudden do you want to walk my horse? Any other time it takes no end of nagging to make you walk her." A look of crafty suspicion set Joan's features into a hard mask, and her eyes narrowed slightly. They were accusing and resentful and suddenly ugly to see, especially because they were the eyes of a mother looking upon her son.

"Jack Dorsey, what do you know about this accident? Come on, now!" And she started shouting: "What did you do to my horse?"

"Ma, I—I didn't mean any harm, honest! I just strung that wire between the barn doorposts for a line to dry our wet bathing suits on. We were playing and running in and out of the barn and the wet suits kept slapping us in the face all the time and getting in our way, so we took the suits down. Well"— obviously his story was becoming harder to tell—"we—we got to fooling around and everybody forgot all about that heavy wire being there. Then we all went out into the field with the horses and I wanted to show everyone how fast Angel could run, so all of us started running. We were whooping and waving, urging Angel to gallop. Then I gave her a smart wallop on her behind and then—" Jack paused in desperation and he continued to talk more slowly, as if measuring every word. "Angel—started—to run. She flew—lickety-split into the barnyard—and smack toward the barn door."

Jack's voice, which was changing due to the newly flowing hormones, began to crack, and "toward the barn door" had squealed out in a high soprano. He raised an arm now, almost as if in supplication, and laying a contrite hand very gently upon the horse's withers, Jack buried his face in the horse's shoulder and wept.

"A lot of good crying is going to do! How could any son of mine do anything so stupid, *stupid?*"

And her son cried harder than ever, for he was being emasculated now by his mother's angry rejection.

"I won't have animals abused!" she barked abusingly at her son. And with righteous indignation she raved on: "I simply will not have any living thing on this farm mistreated!"

It was my guess that it never occurred to Joan how cruelly she was mistreating her own son.

"Joan, shut up! Just shut up. You've done nothing but hold

your head and scream and wail like a banshee this whole damn time!" snapped Ralph, to everyone's surprise.

Even the horse had become upset by Joan's shouting and agitation. When Joan, who was still determined to walk her mare, reached for the animal's bridle, still tirading as she approached, Angel whinnied and reared in the air.

"Enough is enough!" I shouted, churning inside at the turn of events. "Joan, you're too upset and the mare senses it, so why don't you back off and see if you can repair our dinner. After witnessing the result of carelessness and observing the pain and agony Angel has been through, I don't believe there is anything more eloquent you can say to make everybody, adults and *all* children included, feel sorrier or more miserable than we all do now. I believe we've all learned our lesson in the cruelty of 'I forgot' and the danger of 'I didn't think.' So let's all remember this whole scene as a very painful learning experience."

Placing a kind hand on Jack's shoulder, doubtless hoping it would convey a tactile understanding, Ralph said, "C'mon, son. Let's dry and walk the mare together." Already he was working to help his son rebuild his self-respect.

Some people, who really didn't know him, thought Ralph was a henpecked milktoast because of his mild manner, constant congeniality, kindness and downright sweet disposition. They were wrong, I concluded, as I watched Ralph and his son. There walks a secure man, I thought.

"I'll have to tear back to the office, Joe. I've got to get some penicillin and tetanus antitoxin, and replace that horrible hose with a tracheotomy tube. I'll try not to be long."

"I'll fetch a pail of water for the horse and give her a nice cold drink," offered Charlie.

"Oh, no—no! Thanks, anyway, Charlie, but that is the very worst thing we could do; wait until she dries off first and cools down. All we need now is to have the mare come down with colic! We might really lose her then."

When I returned, I noted that no one had eaten much of anything; rather, it looked as if all the adults had poured themselves a good stiff drink or two. Even so, everyone was sitting around kind of subdued. They looked tired and all were sweaty and dirty.

Ralph followed me to the barn and we found Jack still brushing the mare, which was completely dry by now. We cross-tied her in her stall and then I gently removed the garden hose. The procaine had not completely worn off yet and there was no problem with inserting the stainless steel tracheotomy tube and securing it to the skin with several wire sutures. After injecting a dose of penicillin and giving a shot of tetanus antitoxin, we left the horse cross-tied in the stall.

We finally joined the rest of the folks and found the children in the television room, looking like a bouquet of wilted wild flowers, for they had all fallen asleep in careless disarray on the floor. Ralph suggested that we have a nightcap in the living room so we could admire a family portrait they had taken recently, which was hanging in the place of honor over their fireplace.

"Here, look," he said, and pointed proudly to the large gilt-framed photograph.

What I saw was a picture of the entire Dorsey family gathered in front of the huge fireplace in the living room. I had to admit that everybody looked great; even their original cat, Mandy, and their oldest bloodhound, Sleuth, were in the picture. Mandy, the seventeen-year-old cat, did not show her age at all. She was posed demurely, sitting on her haunches with her forepaws placed neatly together in front of her, her tail curled daintily in front and wrapped around her paws. The old cat was looking squarely into the camera, golden eyes smoldering, and each long white whisker, cleaned and fastidiously groomed, showed in sharp contrast against the dark background of little Teddy's black trousers.

And then I came to Sleuth, the bloodhound. . . . I let out a snicker, and then a giggle, which I tried unsuccessfully to squelch.

I guess Joan must have felt insulted, because she asked me what was so damn funny.

"Look at that dog!" I giggled. "Just look at that dog!"

Sleuth was sitting at center stage in the portrait, on the floor along with the children and Mandy. The bloodhound was sitting on his haunches with his left hind leg flexed and tucked under him properly enough, but he had let his right hind leg sag and it was flopped out to the side, exposing his inner thigh. Unfortunately, he had braced his front legs rather far apart, so that his heavy paws provided a frame for his huge, very relaxed scrotum, which was spread out on the floor in front of him, thus exhibiting his two exceedingly large testicles, which looked like a pair of ostrich eggs covered with skin. Once one took a second look at that picture, one never noticed the people anymore, for the eyes were helplessly drawn and glued to the dog's genitals; they dominated the entire portrait!

To this day the portrait hangs in dignity on the wall over the fireplace, the bloodhound's magnificent genitals on continuous display. And over the years that bloodhound has always looked down at us, dolefully perhaps, as only a hound can look, but wonderfully, wonderfully proud.

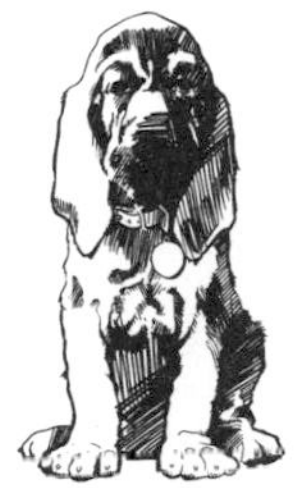

13

I was taught as a student in veterinary gynecology that the best and fastest way to gain a farmer's respect was to be accurate in pregnancy exams.

"Learn to call your shots right," we were instructed. "Nothing vexes a farmer more or embarrasses a veterinarian more than a diagnosis of pregnancy that proves to be mistaken. Do rectal exams at every opportunity, practice, and become skillful in the early diagnosis of pregnancy."

For many reasons, I needed then to gain all the respect I could and therefore did as was suggested. As I look back upon it now, I wonder where I ever found the time to do so many rectal exams. I got so that I could never recognize a cow by her face. The rear end is what the dairy cow is all about; it's all a matter of sex.

Pregnancy diagnosis is one procedure in veterinary medicine that does not require any great strength, but it does require skill. After 120 or 130 days, the fetus of the calf or the foal can be felt through the wall of the rectum, and while one could confuse it with perhaps a firm, large tumor of the mesentery, the diagnosis of pregnancy at that late date is a relatively straightforward procedure. Early diagnosis, however, is a different matter. About three weeks after insemination, if fertilization takes place, you can feel through the wall of the rectum a little lump on one ovary called the corpus luteum, or yellow body. Now, this exam is not as simple as it sounds, for it is not just a question of whether a lump is there or not. The catch is that other lumps, bumps and nodules are frequently present and one must learn to feel the difference and be sure, before announcing that the cow in question is pregnant, that the lump you have felt is in fact a fully developed corpus luteum of pregnancy. One could feel a ripening ovisac, a shriveling atrophied corpus luteum known as a corpus albicans, or even a persistent C.L. that has become cystic. It takes much practice to make a tactile differentiation between all the textures and sizes of the lumps one slips between one's fingers and to come up with consistently correct early pregnancy diagnoses.

Frederick Frye was a tight-lipped, stiff-spined farmer with a bony, protruding Adam's apple that looked like a huge knuckle in the middle of his throat. He was a stern, severe, hard-working man with a no-nonsense attitude toward life. I know for a fact that Mr. Frye resented me the very first time I stepped inside his barn; it was written plainly on his face. He was stuck with me that one time, so to speak, for his usual vet was unavailable and one of his best milkers had a flare-up of acute mastitis. The left rear quarter of the udder looked as if it was ready to explode, it was so hot and swollen, and he figured he had nothing to lose and perhaps maybe a little something to gain by putting up with the likes of a woman for just this one emergency.

Much to the man's surprise and my gratification, this particular cow responded beautifully, and I'd say Mr. Frye was appreciative—grudgingly so, perhaps, but definitely appreciative. He also appreciated all those rectal exams I offered to do on his recently bred cows—for free. I was learning then (I still am, for that matter) and so it was to my advantage to feel as many ovaries as I could, to "train my hands," so to speak. Besides, I did want to gain the farmer's respect and I soon learned that the way to a farmer's heart is through his cow's rectum.

Mr. Frye and I got to understand one another. I found that while he was a pragmatic, drive-a-hard-bargain, old-fashioned farmer who was a little on the know-it-all side, he was not a bigot. He evidently found that I was not afraid of hard work, knew my job, came promptly when called and, above all, was interested and usually cured his cows. He also grew to respect my ability to diagnose pregnancies.

Mr. Frye was really no different than most farmers. While many might have been hesitant at first to try me because I was a newcomer and more especially because I was a woman, their prejudice disappeared as soon as they found that I could cure their animals. That is all they really wanted—someone to cure their animals—and their initial discrimination against a woman in their barn was just due to a preconceived judgment and not to any deep-seated bigotry such as one finds between some races and religions.

Eventually I became Mr. Frye's regular veterinarian, and late one night when I had just finished delivering a calf, he asked a favor of me before I left.

"My hound's been off feed today and looks bloated. I think there's a tumor. Would you quickly feel the belly before you leave and see if you can find anything? Dog's sleeping in the straw—last stall down. I'll fetch a light."

"Never mind, Mr. Frye. I can find my way," and together we walked down the long corridor, for it was a large barn. It was almost pitch black inside the stall, but I could faintly discern the darker form in the straw. The dog got up, yawned and sniffed my hand. I patted its head and talked to it, feeling along the back then to the abdomen, where I placed one hand on either side of the dog. I palpated the abdominal wall in the dark and slipped one, two, three round buoyant masses between my fingers—puppies!

I laughed. "Your hound has three tumors of sorts, Mr. Frye.

This dog is pregnant. As much as seven weeks along, by the feel of things."

"Nep. Not pregnant."

I tried my best to convince him. His Mr. Know-it-all-ness was beginning to show again and I felt a flick of annoyance. It was very late and I was tired. After all my accurate pregnancy diagnoses on his cows, why did he have to be so stubborn now? He had a bee in his bonnet that the dog had a tumor and I couldn't dissuade him.

I sighed in resignation and as we walked back toward the lighted end of the barn, I held out both my hands.

"Mr. Frye, you're arguing with trained, skilled hands—hands that cure the sick. They're precision tools, practically, and they know what they feel."

He studied my hands. "Mebbe so, mebbe so, but I reckon the dog's not pregnant."

"Oh, but it is, Mr. Frye. It is," I said patiently, nodding my head as if to a child.

He pursed his lips. "Wanna bet?"

"I beg your pardon? Bet? You mean a wager?"

"Yep. I'll bet you tonight's fee there's no pups in my dog. I'll pay double fee if I'm wrong." His Adam's apple beckoned to me.

It was much like taking candy from a baby. Mr. Frye was tight with his money and would pinch a nickel until the Indian rode the buffalo. I decided to teach Mr. Know-it-all a lesson.

"You're on," I said. "Do you want me to x-ray the dog or do you want to wait until the pups are born to pay me the extra fee?"

"Nep. No need for all that highfalutin x-ray stuff. Follow me." And he resolutely started back down the corridor again.

"Feel down toward the floor of the belly. Mebbe things will feel different to your trained hands this time."

I felt the dog again to humor him. Three pups, all right,

and I slid my hands around under the abdomen. There was a firm ridge. It felt suspiciously like a penis. Amazingly enough, there were also two testicles. How did *they* get there? I thought to myself. I got up and the two of us walked out to the barnyard.

Mr. Frye looked me in the eye.

"Sorry about your fee." His lips were still in the usual thin, straight line, his eyes expressionless. Deadpan, he was. Only the muscles in his scrawny face twitched, and his Adam's apple wiggled uncontrollably as if it was giggling at me.

I can still hear the nasal twang of his voice as my skilled hands steered the car out of the barnyard.

"If you're willing to deliver the next calf for free, mebbe I'll promise not to tell anybody."

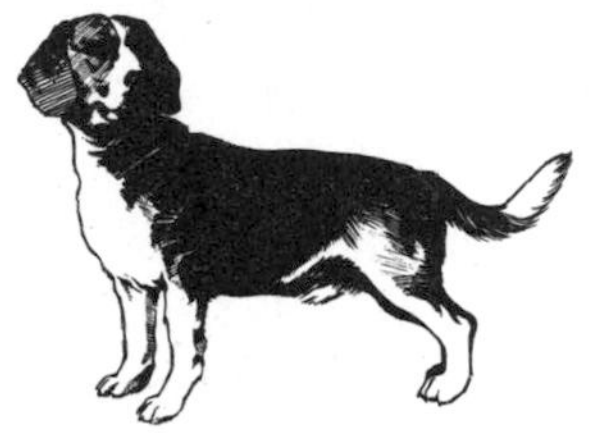

14

It was a warm Saturday afternoon and I was glad that office hours were almost over. We were going to have a dinner party that evening and almost all was in readiness. Mame had cleaned the house all spick-and-span for me and I had prepared most of the food late Friday night after office hours. I was hoping I'd have a few free hours before our guests came for the necessary last-minute preparations.

Just one more person was left in the office. It was Mr. Frye.

"Still off feed. Belly like a pig's." His Adam's apple bobbed in a normal way as he spoke. Neither Mr. Frye nor his Adam's apple made further reference to the episode that had taken place in his barn two evenings before.

I could feel the hard fecal masses butting the end of the rectal thermometer. I palpated the abdomen once again and announced, "What your dog needs, Mr. Frye, is a nice warm, soapy enema! He's just badly constipated, that's all. I can feel the fecal masses—trained hands, you know!"

"Yep. Makes more sense than t'other idea." He didn't bat an eyelash. Mr. Frye left his dog, whose name was Jake, and happily, after a good cleaning out of masses that must have been accumulating for over a week, the dog was right as rain again and eating as eagerly as ever.

I had taken special pains with the dinner. Joe and I were never showoffs, but we did want to put our best foot forward this particular evening. A fellow IBMer, one Andrew Austin, his wife and an English couple were coming to dinner.

Mr. Austin was a distinguished-looking man in his late fifties, handsome in an executive sort of way. His wife was quite stuffy. I remember her tremendous bosom. She was so well endowed that when seated at the table, the poor woman could not see her plate. Every forkful was a suprise as it was brought up to eye level.

"Ah, peas!" we'd hear her say, or "Ah, artichoke hearts!"

The English couple—Tony and Elizabeth Jones—were delightful. Tony was with the English division of the company and he was in the United States on business.

We became acquainted in the living room over a couple of drinks and some hors d'oeuvres, and then we entered the dining room for dinner.

"How charming, simply charming, your table looks, my dear," said the English lady, and she admired my sterling and china.

"Why, thank you, Elizabeth," I said.

I could see Joe beam. He was relaxed and having a good time, for the evening thus far had maintained a cordial, refined and gracious air, which is what Joe wanted. Even the weather was good to us. It was unseasonably warm and pleasant, for spring came early in 1954.

The happy sounds of children's laughter could be heard floating through the dining room windows. Raymond, Marilyn and a group of their friends were still outdoors in the waning spring daylight.

Joe poured the wine, filled with a pleasant sense of well being as he watched Andrew Austin cut into the superbly grilled steak. Just as the man was about to take his first bite, we heard Raymond shout to his friends and his words came very audibly to our ears.

"Come on, everybody," he yelled. "Let's all play torsion of the uterus!"

The fork stopped and remained suspended in midair.

As I've related, Joe's brown eyes have a way of changing color. His countenance remained serene, but his eyes darkened. They weren't even a dark brown; they were jet black, black with anger, and how they flashed! Dart! Snap!

There followed wild shouts of glee from the children and much laughter as they all started to roll down the grassy hill that could be seen from the dining room.

"Torsion of the uterus?" asked Tony, with a twinkle in his eye. "Never heard of that game before. Sounds a bit interesting, to say the least—eh?"

There followed a painful silence.

I chewed on my beef.

From the time Joe and I were first married, I learned not to discuss my work when we were in the company of others. Joe hated to spend an evening talking about animals. If anyone ever did ask me a question about my work, I would answer as politely and briefly as possible and immediately divert the conversation to something else, like flying or sports—anything but animals.

"Will you please explain our son's remark, Jeanne?" Joe asked stiffly.

I swallowed my mouthful of steak.

"A pregnant cow," I began, "can sometimes have its uterus twisted upon itself—that is, a revolution of the organ upon its long axis. It can be a 180-degree revolution and sometimes a complete revolution of 360 degrees. In fact, there are cases recorded in which there were *two* complete turns of the gravid uterus. Try to picture a hammock twisted and slung around on itself and you can begin to get the idea. Anyway, the way we treat such cases, to unsling the uterus, is to roll the cow over. You can determine which way the uterus has flipped by looking into the vagina of the cow. When the cow has a torsion, the vaginal walls are twisted into spiral folds and the direction of these folds indicates the direction of the torsion. It helps to have a hill to roll the cow down, and when our son heard this he thought it hilariously funny. The children never just roll down grassy hills anymore; they play 'torsion of the uterus.' "

"Fantastic!" exclaimed Andrew Austin.

His wife, aghast, said, "I never heard of any treatment so crude."

"It is crude." Joe started talking now, having decided to join the conversation rather than fight it with silence. "I saw Jeanne treat a cow with this problem once. Christ, with all the farmhands scurrying around, and Jeanne shouting orders and trying to be heard over the bellowing of the cow, it was like a Chinese fire drill, rolling that cow down the hill. They had to roll the poor beast over seven times in order to completely reduce the displacement."

"I had no idea," said Andrew's wife, shuddering, "that veterinary medicine could be so—so primitive! Jeanne, did you *really* roll a pregnant cow down a hill?"

"Absolutely." I couldn't help laughing at her disbelief. "Not only did the cow survive the gymnastics, but she carried to term and calved normally!"

"My word! I'd like to see my gynecologist try to do that to me when I'm pregnant!" Elizabeth laughed.

"He'd probably never have to," I explained, "because you are not prone to torsion of the uterus. You stand upright on two feet and when you are pregnant, your uterus and fetus are cradled in your pelvis, like resting in a basin. Your cervix and vagina are compressed, whereas with a four-legged animal, the pregnant or gravid uterus slumps because of gravity toward the diaphragm, and the weight of the uterus is suspended from the perineum through the vagina and vulva—like the hammock again. You all might think the procedure in reducing a torsion of the uterus in a cow is crude, but it is mechanically sound in principle, and what's most important, it works. The cow would die if not treated, for the torsion twists the blood vessels so as to cut off the circulation, and strangulation of the uterus would be the result."

"We have had horses all our lives, just outside Winchester, and we never had any problem like this," Tony remarked.

"I believe that," I answered. "Interestingly, a horse habitually rolls itself over on the ground and yet torsion of the uterus in the mare is very rare. On the other hand, a cow never rolls, yet torsion is common in the cow. No one really knows what causes torsion of the uterus. Maybe it's the way the cow gets up—you know, hind end first, so that the uterus is completely suspended for a moment. Perhaps this is what favors torsion—I don't know. I doubt if anyone else knows, either, why the cow is most prone to this problem."

"You folks think that's crude," said Joe, giving up all pretense of even trying to maintain a genteel table conversation. "You should see what they do to a cow that has bloat. Sometimes fermentation in a cow's rumen, or first stomach, gets out of hand and tremendous pressures build up which can rupture the wall of the rumen if the pressure isn't relieved. To relieve this pressure, they puncture, actually puncture, the cow's abdominal wall—through the skin, muscles and peritoneum, and finally through the wall of the rumen itself. They puncture with a hollow-tubed trocar and the gas escapes through the inserted tube."

"My lord!" Andrew's wife again, and she glared at me as if she planned to notify the local ASPCA.

"The gas formed by the fermentation of ensilage in the cow's rumen is practically pure methane—CH_4." I tried to dignify the procedure by throwing in a smattering of chemistry, to make things sound more scientific.

But Joe wouldn't let it alone now, and he threw discretion to the winds by adding, "When this gas escapes from the cow, you can actually light the gas as it comes out the end of the tube and the methane will burn with a pretty blue flame. The cow will just stand there with a little gas burner flaming at her side. I've seen Jeanne do this. Impresses the hell out of the farmer."

"By Jove!" The Englishman laughed in disbelief. "Whatever would you do if the bloody thing backfired?"

I could have kissed the man; his comment broke the ice. We all laughed hilariously now. Andy's wife's bosom quivered, reminding me of an earth tremor, she was laughing so. When I was able to talk, I said, "You know, Tony, the most amusing thing of all to me is that your comment happens to be one of my old professor's favorite jokes! He told it during every lecture on the treatment of bloat that was ever delivered to every veterinary student since the beginning of time!"

Tony had another laugh, then shook his head, saying, "And I thought for a moment that I was so witty and original!"

The big bosom was still quivering, and then we heard about a gay discovery.

"Ah! A ripe olive!"

The evening ended; they had gone home; but all was not as well as it seemed. Despite all the hilarity and laughter, Joe was very unhappy about the main topic of conversation throughout dinner, which he felt was very uncouth.

"I work my balls off," he scolded as we were preparing for bed, "to provide a comfortable home, decent furniture, cars, an airplane. Can't you get it through your head that I'm trying to raise a well-mannered family and maintain a well-run household? No matter how hard I try, I can't seem to ever have anything go right around here. Like this evening." He was standing in his socks and underwear now, hanging his trousers carefully on a hanger. "I wanted just one lousy evening to be gracious and dignified, and what happens? Torsion of the uterus!"

I started to say, "I'm sorry," but I never got the chance.

"Torsion of the uterus. My ass! I was so mad at that table, I would have sold that practice of yours for a plug nickel to the first bum who came to the door." He took his undershirt off and threw it in disgust on the floor. Savagely he tore off the left sock, then the right. The way he pulled at them was the way skin is pulled down the leg in some accident cases I've seen. Next, he pulled his undershorts down, sat on the edge of the bed, pulled them over his feet and threw them clear across the room. They hit the wall, started falling, but were caught by the corner of a picture frame. I don't know where that picture ever came from. There was a sad Little Lord Fauntleroy type of lad in it, I remember. He looked doomed as he was packed off in a horse and carriage with his valise and humpback trunk. It was entitled "Black Monday, or The Return to School."

Just as I thought the tirade had ended, Joe was off again.

"Another thing that was in very poor taste this evening. I noticed you weren't wearing your wedding ring. Christ! I have to work with these people, Jeanne. What are they going to think?" There was a painful pause. "Well? What have you got to say for yourself?"

I had so hoped Joe would not notice the ring was missing, but I should have known better. Nothing ever escapes Joe Logue.

"I lost it, kind of."

"Lost it?" Joe bellowed. "Jesus H. Christ! How could you be so careless? An item as important as a *wedding ring!*"

For years now Joe hadn't worn his wedding ring. He had

mentioned very casually, many years ago, that since he was an electrical engineer it could be dangerous for him to wear anything metal on his fingers. I always thought it a rather lame excuse, and felt that whether Joe consciously realized it or not, that ring somehow symbolized to him a ring through the nose. I never said anything, never paid it any mind, as a matter of fact, although I thought it interesting that I should think of it now.

I waved my ringless left hand in a weary gesture. "Look, Joe, let's not make this ring episode any worse than it is. If you could only have been there!" and I tried to explain. "You see, I had never been to the Wassenmuellers' farm before. They are a couple right from the old country and I thought the man would faint when he first saw me. 'Vere iss your husbant?' was what I was greeted with. I told him you were at work and I almost felt sorry for the poor soul when he finally got it through his head that *I* was the doctor. He struck his forehead with the palm of his hand and kept repeating, *'Gott in Himmel.'* He kept shaking his head in disbelief, all the while peering vainly into the car, hoping that there would be a *real* vet tucked away in the back seat somewhere. When his wife came on the scene there were more *Gott in Himmel*s, and I could see from the way her apron kept convulsing that she was wringing her hands like mad under it. Joe, can't you just imagine what that did to my ego and self-confidence? So please, let us have no more tirades now.

"Anyway, I had to deliver a calf. Thank heavens that went smoothly. And *now* we come to the ring. Whoever packed my bag forgot to pack my obstetrical glove, so I had to deliver bare-armed, and what with the tight fit between the calf, the cow's pelvis and my fingers, and all that lubrication—well, the ring just slid off as I pulled my hand out with the calf! I didn't notice the ring was missing until I got home to a waiting room full of people. They all helped me look for the ring, and when I finally realized where it must be, inside that cow, I sneaked off to the back room so no one could hear me as I phoned the Wassenmuellers. I told them to tie the cow so when she cleaned they could retrieve my ring. Their only comment was *'Gott in Himmel,'* but sure enough, they poked around and found it! They gave the ring to the GLF man and I can get it from him downtown on Monday. That will save gas and an extra trip way out to their farm." I tried to end my explanation with a bright, efficient smile. This really did not help at all. The cloud over our heads was blacker now than the Fauntleroy lad's Black Monday.

"That is absolutely repulsive!" stormed Joe. "One disgusting episode after another! Jesus H. Christ! Isn't this awful!" Joe got between the sheets in a huff, and lay like a huge, silent log, his back to me.

Contritely I crawled into bed, kept my hands to myself and my mouth shut, and quietly endured.

The next morning Joe still hadn't cooled off. To make matters worse, I had a horse to castrate and planned to leave right after breakfast.

"What a way for a wife of mine to spend a Sunday morning," he bristled. "Remember!" And he wagged a finger under my nose. "No standing castrations! Throw the son of a bitch and truss him up good. All I need is to come home and find your head's been kicked in. I'm telling you, Jeanne, it's a dangerous business, yours. Dangerous!" He dismissed his empty plate by pushing it away from him with a vicious shove, as though the plate somehow was to blame.

The children ate their breakfast in silence; they knew when to keep their mouths shut.

"Remember that insurance agent?" Joe ranted as he threw down his napkin. "Wouldn't insure you, right?" *Bam!* He pounded the table. "Why wouldn't he insure you?" *Bam!*

"Because your work is too dangerous, that's why!" He pushed his chair from the table. "I'm pissed! Real pissed!"

And the Red Baron was off. He jammed his goggled flying helmet on his head and, scarf flying, went off to get away from it all and relax in the PT22, his experimentally licensed airplane which was all set up for aerobatics, complete with an inverted fuel system so that he could fly it upside down.

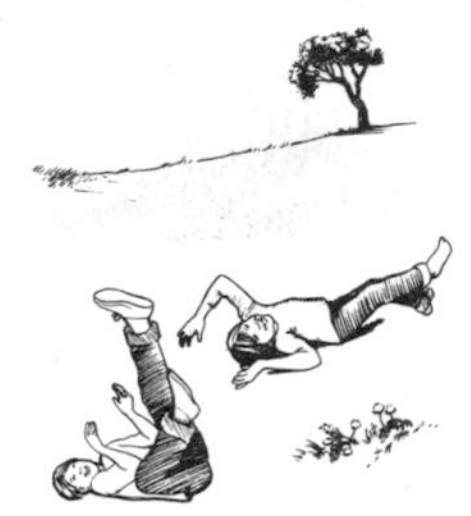

15

I figured that my husband had a legitimate gripe. Our life style was out of the ordinary, to say the least, and I began to try even harder to make things nice for him and to take greater pains with my personal appearance. I fussed with my hair more and tried to let my nails grow longer and keep them all the same length. I even used nail polish on weekends. Small endeavors, perhaps, but my intentions were noble. Yet despite my efforts, it seemed for a while that no matter how I tried, I was doomed to get into trouble.

It was New Year's Eve and we were going to have a party. The lights on the outdoor Christmas tree cast nuances of color on the smooth, unruffled snow, which was fine and dry and granular, giving the ground a mat finish like the sheen of the wrong side of madras satin.

The interior of the refrigerator was also a kaleidoscope of color. I had made salads decorated with bright-red poinsettia flowers which I had cut out of pimentos, with leaves fashioned from smooth, firm green peppers. Shrimp were clustered in pink ringlets and variegated red-and-white roses bloomed where the radishes lay.

I was dressed in a well-fitted bright new outfit, high heels and dangly earrings. I made sure that my nails were polished, and that my hair, shampooed and shining, was arranged attractively. I must have looked good to Joe, because he kissed me and whispered, "You look beautiful. This is the way I like to see you look." I felt deliciously feminine for a change, and was happy because Joe was happy.

The guests had all arrived and everybody was in a carefree, festive mood. Joe and I were dancing; we were all going to have a blast.

It was in the middle of "Chattanooga Choo-Choo" that we heard the phone.

"I won't be long, Joe. I'll be back in time to sing 'Auld Lang Syne.' "

"Jesus H. Christ! Not on New Year's Eve?"

"Yes, a horse with colic on New Year's Eve. There is no question but what I have to go. Mr. Hurley says the animal is rolling and groaning—just out of its mind with the pain."

All my pretty things were put aside, as I climbed into my large-animal clothes. I donned a heavy jacket, pulled on a pair of boots, tied a kerchief under my chin and said a few hasty goodbyes to the guests.

I gave Mr. Hurley's horse some chloral hydrate to relieve his pain and quiet him enough so that I could pass a stomach tube. A good bit of pressure was relieved through this and while the tube was in place, I gave him an antiferment and some mineral oil. I was relieved to find upon rectal exam that there was no volvulus or impaction, and that it seemed to be a case of simple flatulant colic—if any case of colic can be considered simple. Already the horse had stopped groaning and straining and kicking at his flanks. I reminded Mr. Hurley to get the horse dry, as he was still wet with perspiration, and to keep walking him.

I had made good time—it was still a bit before midnight. As I was about to leave, Mr. Hurley said, "While you're still here, and since it won't take but a few minutes, would you check this one cow for me before you go? She was bred about a month ago; can you tell me if she's pregnant?"

I couldn't very well say no to so small a request, so I put on a glove, and with a manicured hand, I lifted aside the tail like a curtain and inserted my arm up the cow's rectum. I found the right ovary and felt of it carefully—smooth, slightly oval, resilient and firm. I felt for the left one, and there it was, the raised nodule centrally placed on the ovary—the corpus luteum of pregnancy.

I was about to withdraw my arm when it happened. There was not one peristaltic ripple of warning—just a sudden convulsion and a giant brown geyser shot out of that cow like Old Faithful. It blew me out of the rectum and jet-propelled me across the barn. The stream seemed to follow me like a huge fire hose—into my hair, my face, forcing its way around my neck and behind my ears and trickling down my thoroughly saturated shirt. I could feel the glop run down my brassiere straps, hesitate like water on the continental divide and then flow around the mounds and pour down on either side. It was awful—just awful! I thought of my pretty hairdo and my party dress.

I looked at Mr. Hurley through manure-mascaraed lashes. I hated him. If he had so much as looked like a smile, I would have killed him. His shirt was clean and his sleeves were buttoned at his wrists. He even had a tie on! The most maddening thing, for some reason, was his hair. It was combed and neatly parted, clean and very curly. Curly Hurley, I thought, as I glared at him through my peculiar mud pack. I was sorry his cow was pregnant; I wished I could have had bad news for him.

But Curly Hurley did not smile. He rolled up his shirt sleeves and heavily starched cuffs smartly, got a stick of sorts and tried to scrape me down. He took one last look at the offending cow, shrugged, and stated matter-of-factly, "Something she et, no doubt."

We lined the front seat of my car with newspapers. I climbed stickily behind the wheel and drove away.

I simply did not know what to do. I could not enter the house in my present state of attire and I couldn't take all my clothes off in the vestibule and scamper naked through the house headed toward the shower, for all those people would still be there. No one must see me this way! No one! I couldn't bear it. Better they all believed that I never got back before they left.

I hid the car in a neighbor's driveway, scurried through our backyard and crouched under a living room window. I was just in time to see everyone counting: Nine! Eight! Seven! The ball was once again falling on Times Square and they were all counting together: Six! Five! Four!

Star sensed something and put her nose against the window opposite mine. Even my own dog didn't recognize me. She gave a menacing growl, but no one paid any attention. I crawled to the dining room side of the house, which afforded a view of the stairway, hoping perhaps I could dash madly up the stairs undetected and make it into the sanctuary of the bathroom while no one was looking. Unfortunately, I was trapped, for there was a couple at the foot of the stairway. They were chanting: Three! Two! One! and they started kissing Happy New Year. They almost seemed disgusting. Everyone looked so warm and happy and here I was, poor me, cold and miserable.

Strands of my manure-encrusted hair were being whipped by the wind and they twisted and twined around on each other, forming thick, ropy coils which began to freeze into Medusa-like snakes. I crept to the kitchen window. There they were, all milling about, laughing like idiots and taking all my good food from my refrigerator. I didn't dare to lick my lips, but my, that food looked good and I was starving. I could hear Guy Lombardo's music in the background.

Nobody seemed the least bit worried about me. I felt very

sorry for myself and I had good reason. I took the key to the boarding kennel from its hook, walked out back and let myself inside the heated kennel house. The dogs started barking, but quieted down a moment later when I told them all to be quiet.

I curled up in a large empty kennel, pulled some straw bedding around me and tried to sleep.

Finally I heard engines starting and cars beginning to roll out of the parking area. At last they were all gone, thank God.

"It's about time!" I fumed as I made a dash to the house.

Joe must have heard me come in, for he called down to me from upstairs, "Where the shit have you been all night?"

I was in the shower for over half an hour. I scrubbed and rinsed and scrubbed and rinsed. Then, in my bathrobe and with a towel turbaned around my thoroughly shampooed hair, I started to clean the mess left from the party. I crawled into bed at six thirty-five in the morning.

In a sense I was lucky, for the phone didn't ring that morning until ten minutes past eight.

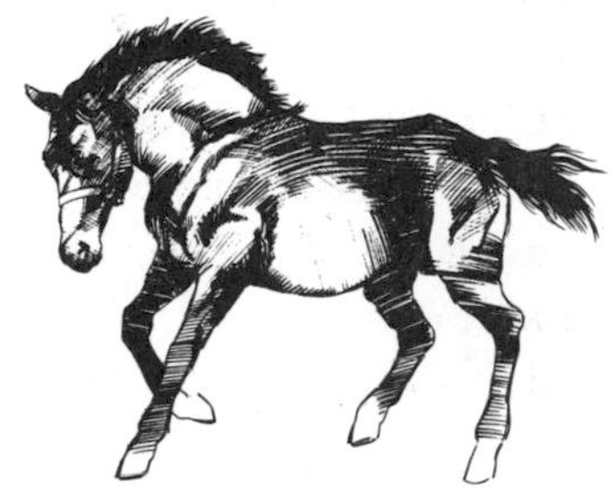

16

It seemed that I was damned if I didn't and damned if I did. If my appearance was one to be criticized on New Year's Eve, it was criticized with venom again the following weekend, but this time I was dressed—very nicely dressed!

I had returned from a small horse farm near Bearsville which had a number of nice hunter horses. The stables were owned by a Mrs. Broome, whom I had never met, this having been my first call to attend any of her horses.

Unfortunately, one of her fine animals was suffering from periodic ophthalmia, an inflammatory disease of the eye which in advanced stages involves not only the iris, but the lens, retina and vitreous body. Eventually this causes blindness—"moon blindness," the old-timers called it, perhaps because of its periodicity in the onset of symptoms. The attacks frequently occurred in near monthly cycles, making them think that the onset had something to do with the changes in the moon.

The horse's eye was in the advanced stages and I felt great pity for him as in agony he turned the inflamed eye away from the light.

"The eye is doomed," I told the caretaker. "I'll treat the eye if you wish and I'll give the poor horse something to relieve the pain—but as far as saving the eye, it's hopeless. There is little or no sight left in the eye at all now. The eyeball has already atrophied and you can see that the lens is opaque. See how the pupil is locked into a closed position from all the scar tissue and adhesions that have formed? It's a sick, unhealthy, ulcerated eye, and to keep it in the horse's head is a very real source of potential danger to the entire horse."

"Is there nothing you can do to save it? Are you sure?" The man gave his woolen scarf an extra turn around his neck and jammed his hands despondently back into his pockets.

"I'm sorry. There's nothing I can do and I'm very sure. You know as well as I do how many times this eye must have been treated. You can see it's just gone from bad to worse. It ought to be enucleated—in fact, it should have been removed before this. I'm surprised it was left in so long. Keeping it is only prolonging an agony, and I can guarantee that it's only a matter of time before the other eye becomes involved."

"The boss won't like what you have to say."

"I don't blame her. I don't like it either. I'm sorry for the horse, but his eye cannot be saved."

The caretaker chewed his thumbnail for a moment, as though this helped him think more clearly. He suggested that I treat the animal as best I could and that when he saw his boss he'd tell her what I had told him.

I injected the horse with streptomycin and told the man that if the owner insisted on treating the horse instead of operating on it, the injections would have to be repeated daily for at least five days.

"There will be another attack no matter how we treat it, but at least this may give the horse some relief for a short time." I instilled an ophtalmic solution containing prednisone, a new drug which was proving of great benefit in reducing inflammatory processes.

As I left, I suggested a dark stall for the animal's comfort and added that Mrs. Broome should feel free to call me if she had any questions.

As soon as I returned home, I showered and started dressing. We were on our way to a dinner which was a quasi-business affair and as usual we were pressed for time. It was Joe's turn in the shower and while he was getting ready, I filed a few rough edges from my nails and applied a fresh coat of nail polish. I wanted to look nice for Joe to make up for the New Year's Eve debacle.

My heart sank as I heard a car pull snappily into the driveway and come to an abrupt halt. I could hardly afford another social conflict again so soon. It really was not fair to Joe, but then, that shingle was still hanging out front, so I resolutely went to answer the door, holding my fingertips carefully so I wouldn't smudge my nail polish. I opened the door, reeking of banana oil.

A woman stepped into the vestibule, sniffed the air and eyed me from head to toe with frank disapproval.

"Hmph!" she snorted. "Go and tell that person who calls himself a doctor of veterinary medicine that Mrs. Broome wants a few words with him!" She planted the tip of her black umbrella, almost puncturing the floor in front of her feet, and rested both hands firmly on the curved wooden handle. She had short, boyishly bobbed straight hair, and wore a square wool tweed suit, dark lisle stockings and flat-heeled heavy oxfords. She was Mrs. Business herself.

"I'm that person, Mrs. Broome. I'm Dr. Logue."

"You! You?" She spoke as if I were the embodiment of a sacrilege, a living profanity, a desecration to my profession. "*You're* the one who wants to remove my horse's eye? Look at you—what could you possibly know? *Look at you!*" She was almost screaming at me as she pointed accusingly a short, square, shaking finger under my nose.

I looked down at myself and I had to admit that compared

to Mrs. Broome, I looked like Zsa Zsa Gabor.

"Why did they ever let something like *you* into the veterinary college—at Cornell, no less! Look at you!" She spat each word. "What could you possibly know? You don't even look like a veterinarian. You look like—you look like—like something that belongs in a *chorus line!"* She shook her head as though she had uttered a foul mouthful.

Now, if anybody said that to me today, I'd take ten dollars off his or her bill, but as I look back on the moment, I recall that I felt insulted. Her remark didn't bother me too much, really. I was a bit amused, but mostly insulted.

Then, to my alarm, she began losing her composure to a degree that was unwarranted by the situation. After all, I had only treated her horse properly and given my honest opinion.

She was red in the face, quaking like an aspen in the wind. I sensed she was not so much preoccupied with her horse anymore and suddenly realized that I was the direct and sole object of her rage.

In front of my very eyes, she disintegrated and became completely irrational. The more I think of it, "unglued" is a very good description of her.

"You're not a vet!" she screamed, and commenced to belt me on my head and around my ears with her pocketbook, which looked like the Pony Express's original mail bag. "You're not! You're not!"

I dodged the next blow and managed to disarm her.

Raymond tore into the room at the sound of the commotion, placed himself between the two of us and pushed Mrs. Broome away from me.

Marilyn stood wide-eyed at the kitchen door, taking everything in with a bewildered silence.

"A chorus girl! A chorus girl!" Mrs. Broome choked, livid with rage.

Together, Raymond and I managed to get her out of the office and point her toward her car.

"You had better go home, Mrs. Broome, and seriously consider visiting a psychiatrist. I say this as a helpful suggestion and not as a slur—you need psychiatric help."

I tried to repair my hairdo with trembling fingers. I had never been the object of such hatred before, and I must admit it upset me.

"Daddy! Daddy!" shouted Marilyn. "A lady just told Mother to join a chorus line!"

"You all right, Ma?" Raymond looked worried and yet he sounded very protective. He suddenly looked very grown up to me and I wondered how I had ever hatched anything so wonderful.

"I'm fine, Ray—really. Thanks!" I smiled at him.

He put an arm around my waist and we headed toward the kitchen door.

"Well"—he gave a chuckle—"that Mrs. Broome sure made a clean sweep!"

I had to laugh and it relaxed me. A child who makes his parent laugh! As we stepped together through the door into our home, I counted a very special blessing.

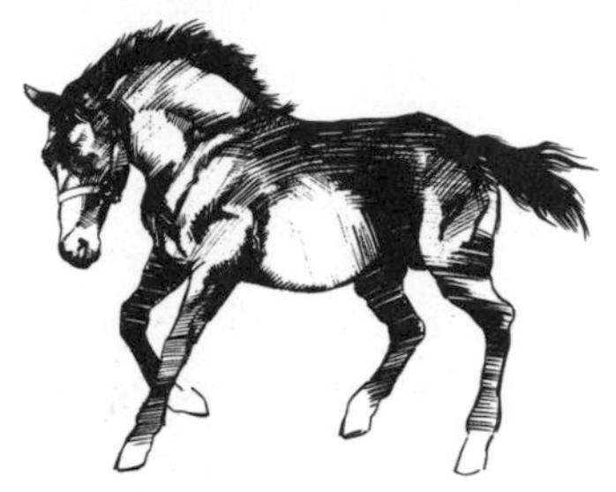

17

From the surgery window I could see Raymond working out back, cleaning the boarding-kennel runs. Ray loved our dog, Star, very much and accorded every pet that was placed in our care the same careful attention he'd want his own dog to receive if she were boarded elsewhere. Ray was the best kennel man any vet ever had, for he kept the runs really clean. All wastes were removed promptly and any residue or urine was thoroughly hosed away with a strong blast from the hose nozzle. I can remember thinking at just that moment how much I loved him, but then it was time to remove the mother's hat and don the doctor's. My family faded from my mind as I anesthetized the first patient of the day with an injection of Nembutal in the little back room that was my surgery.

Some of my happiest hours were spent in that room. There was a quiet serenity about the brightly lighted cubicle, and usually the only audible sounds were the slow, steady breathing of the unconscious animal, and clear metallic sounds such as the staccato *click-click-click* as hemostats and forceps were clamped shut, or the clear clink of an instrument as it was discarded into a gleaming stainless steel pan. There was today one other sound, and that one perhaps was the most authoritative of all. It was a series of clear short whistles, the call of the cardinal perched on a bough of the crab apple tree growing outside the surgery window.

I worked alone in contented solitude. The schedule promised a light work load today. There were just two abscess cases and one cruciate ligament to repair in a dog's knee. I planned to do the joint surgery first and leave the abscesses—what I called "dirty" surgery—till last. I loved bone surgery because it was such a positive type of repair work, not a destructive effort such as a spay operation or a castration. Every time I opened a knee joint I imagined that I was crawling inside a living sea shell, with gleaming surfaces all about. Such smooth, curved perfection! Sometimes, as a result of the injury, I saw osteophytes, little buttonlike bits of cancellous bone which would grow along the margin of the joint, and they would look to me like a string of tiny coalesced pearls. I looked forward to the day when technology was advanced enough so someone could develop an artificial prosthetic joint for the knee, the most complex joint in the body.

I finished making a new ligament from a strip of fascia from the dog's thigh, repaired the knee and got on to the first abscess operation. The little silver toy poodle was very lethargic, had had a poor appetite and also some daily vomiting for the past two weeks. I could not imagine why the owners had not brought him in sooner. It was the swelling which appeared on the dog's left side—an abscess which had increased in size rather rapidly—that finally induced the owner to bring the dog in. More than a cupful of creamy custardlike pus oozed from the incision. On and on it drained in a never-diminishing flow, a poisonous shade of green. "*Pseudomonas pyocyaneus,* the bacillus of green pus." I could still hear Professor Hagan's voice at Cornell.

As the abscess drained, the ballonlike swelling under the skin became deflated, and after the cushion effect of the fluid was gone, I felt a hard object. A piece of wood? Or wire? No, it could not be wire; it felt too blunt. I started enlarging the incision to thoroughly clean the area and establish drainage. And then I saw it—a Popsicle stick! But there was something odd about the thing—the end of it was so round and smooth. How could it possibly have penetrated the skin? Certainly, if a blunt object had managed to penetrate, it would have torn the skin and left a very noticeable wound, one that even the most careless pet owner would have noticed. This was no shaggy outdoor farm dog. It was a house pet, a lap dog, no less. The owners surely would have noticed a wound had there been one. Puzzled, I reached in with a pair of forceps to lift the stick out, but it would not budge. I got a firmer grip and gently tried to remove the Popsicle stick, but it held fast, anchored, it seemed, to the muscles of the abdominal wall. I should have thought that it would have remained free, floating around in all that pea soup, rather than adhering to the muscle wall at right angles.

It took almost a minute before I fully realized what it was. I stood staring, not believing my eyes. Before me was the smooth, rounded end of the ice cream stick with almost two inches of the stick exposed. It protruded straight out from the abdominal wall because the Popsicle stick had arrived where it was now from the *inside!*

Incredulously I gently palpated the poodle's abdomen. The anesthetic caused good muscle relaxation, and almost immediately I felt the other end of the stick through the body wall and I moved it a bit. Sure enough, the exposed end moved slightly. With comprehension came wonder that the dog was still alive.

And so I opened him up, this fragile toy poodle, which somehow had survived for at least two weeks with a shaft of wood piercing his body. There must have been a lot of straining and retching over the past weeks, and why the stomach had not ruptured and the dog had not died of peritonitis I'll never know. A miraculous role had been played by the omentum, that double sheet of connecting peritoneum. The maze of mesenteries, rich in lymphatics, like a motile lacy doily, had moved to the precise spot where the stick had eroded through the stomach wall and had shrouded the area with a veil of lymphocytes. As the stick worked its way out of the stomach, the omentum enveloped it, preventing infection from breaking through to the rest of the peritoneal cavity. Moving slowly, like the hour hand of a clock, and covered with omentum, the stick had worked its way to the dog's left, past the spleen, until it butted against the sheet of parietal peritoneum which lines the inside of the abdominal wall. A little tunnel of defensive white cells had formed over the entire distance between the hole in the stomach and the hole made at the point of exit from the peritoneal cavity. There were no signs of infection; the cavity was clean and as good as gold!

After piercing the peritoneum, the stick had pressed against the innermost muscle supporting the abdominal wall, the transverse abdominal muscle. The next barrier had been the internal oblique, and then the external oblique, and finally the large cutaneous muscle of the trunk. One by one, at each point where the blunt end of the Popsicle stick had pressed, a small area of necrosis had formed, the tissue had liquefied, and the stick had been propelled on through. The stick completed its passage by erupting just behind the thirteenth rib, and finally it formed a large abscess under the skin. I wondered whether if I had not intervened, nature could have completed the job all by herself. I sensed that peculiar feeling of reverence once again, the reverence I always feel when I see nature quietly performing complex little miracles.

The surprise inside the toy poodle caused the operation to take longer than I had expected, but I was finally ready for the third dog, a nice little beagle hound. I anticipated a rapid conclusion—for this time it *was* only an abscess—until another unexpected turn of events presented itself. Just as I was pulling off my surgical gloves, the beagle stopped breathing! The heartbeat was regular and strong, and I gave immediate artificial respiration to keep the dog alive.

Darn! The dog had seemed so perfectly anesthetized and everything went so smoothly.

I kept up the rhythmical compression of the dog's rib cage and then the sudden release of my hands, first pressing the air out and then letting fresh air flow back in when the ribs were allowed to spring back into place. I rested a moment, but the dog did not start breathing. I gave mouth-to-mouth resuscitation until I got out of breath and had to resume working his ribs in and out with my hands. "Out comes the bad air, in goes the good air"—in and out, in and out. I injected an amphetamine to stimulate the breathing reflex. In and out, in and out, I kept kneading his ribs. Over two hours had gone by. Every time I paused to see if the dog could take a breath of air, I held my own breath in anxious expectation until I thought my lungs would burst. Cautiously I gave a second dose of amphetamine and continued with the artificial respiration. I could hear cars coming and going in the driveway and I imagined that the pet owners in the waiting room had got tired of waiting and were going home. The heartbeat was still full and strong, and to my amazement now the beagle started to shiver and quiver, sure signs of an animal coming out of anesthesia. Surely now he *must* start breathing! But no. The dog still could not breathe. I continued breathing for him. The anesthesia began wearing off faster now and soon the dog's eyes opened. He blinked, looked right at me and started to move around a bit, *but he still could not breathe!* Even when the dog became fully awake his respiratory center remained paralyzed! I was horrified! I could see panic in the animal's eyes. Every time I stopped giving the poor dog artificial respiration to see if the breathing center in his brain would take over, the fear-stricken creature would turn his face to me with the most pathetic imploring look in his soulful brown eyes. I was sweating now and out of breath from empathetic suspension of my own breathing as I waited for the dog to take a breath on his own. I started talking to him to try to comfort him, encouraging him to breathe. I had to rest my arms once more. How could this be happening? Why of all the dogs I ever anesthetized did this particular animal's respiratory center become so completely paralyzed by the Nembutal? I kept hoping his carbon dioxide buildup would trigger the breathing reflex. How long could this go on? I was just about to resume the pumping when I heard a faltering intake of air! The dog expelled it and after what seemed like an eternity a second breath was taken, then a third and a fourth and a fifth. An enormous sigh of relief escaped from me. I could see the look of blessed relief in the dog's face as he half closed his eyes and sucked that sweet air into himself. I hugged him to me and rocked him back and forth in my arms as I would a baby and the beagle squirmed happily and licked my cheek and my ear. My, how I loved that little dog!

I promised myself that if the medical supply houses ever produced anything like an anesthesia machine with new volatile anesthetic gases other than ether—and I knew they were working on this—I would be first in line to buy one.

The next day the silver toy poodle ate, with relish, his first decent meal in weeks and kept it down. He made a speedy and uneventful recovery and the only souvenir of the Popsicle stick episode was the change in the color of his fur at the site of his operation. For some reason, instead of silver, the fur that grew in was almost black. But the little beagle was not quite over the trauma of his spooky ordeal. Poor dog, he remained timid and frightened for several days, but gradually his self-confidence returned and he regained his merry heart.

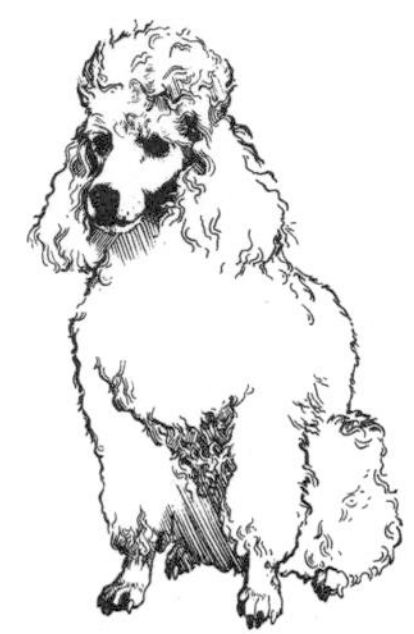

18

"You've probably heard people say this before, Dr. Logue," said Mrs. Rousseau, "but honestly, this cat behaves more like a dog than a cat. I hate to think of spaying her, but we can't stand the tomcat fights night after night anymore, and the way Sheba writhes in agony! I keep thinking she must be in pain, and I simply can't bear to watch her. I thought she was having a convulsion the first time I saw her act that way. Remember how panic-stricken I was when I brought her in to you? I was afraid she'd die! I never knew some cats could carry on so just from being in heat. It's gotten so now Sheba's in heat continuously. My lord! The caterwauling! Now I know where the term 'cathouse' must have originated. The strange thing is that though Sheba attracts the males and drives them crazy, and she's obviously in heat, she won't permit them to try to breed with her."

"Sheba has probably developed cysts on her ovaries, Mrs. Rousseau, and isn't ovulating normally," I explained. "When the pituitary gland fails to produce enough luteinizing hormone, large cystic follicles form on the ovaries, which produce estrogens and cause the persistent symptoms of heat, like nymphomania. Sheba is well named," I added, stroking the cat. "A mature female cat is called a queen, while the mature male is the tom."

"My Sheba a nymphomaniac! Tell me something, do males ever have this problem?"

"Yes, they may experience satyriasis, due to lack of exercise, frustration and boredom, or sometimes from a disease of the penis. Anyway, there's a disturbance of the libido center in the brain. The main symptoms are masturbation and an abnormal sexual awareness. Satyriasis is more frequent in dogs than in cats, though," I informed her.

"It sure sounds complicated—all those hormones."

"I agree. The interplay, interdependence and series of checks and balances between all the numerous endocrine glands is a very complex bit of physiology. Let one little thing go wrong—just one aberrant gland can upset the whole apple cart!"

I had continued to stroke Sheba as we talked, and she had become sexually stimulated. Her tail quivered, straight in the air, and she started a rhythmical kneading motion of her paws.

"Has Sheba had any personality changes? Cats with this problem frequently become very irritable and nervous—sometimes even vicious."

"Sheba *has* become nervous, but I've never seen her nasty. Never attempts to scratch or bite us. The only time I see her fight like a spitfire is with the toms recently. She got out by accident—a terrible time. She wouldn't let them near her! We always wanted one of her kittens, she's such a nice cat. I just hate to have her spayed."

"Sheba is sterile in her present condition, but if you want to try to save her for breeding, we could try injecting gonadotropin. To tell you the truth, though, this method is usually not very successful. Spaying is the best procedure."

"I do hope she'll be all right. I know you advise that an animal shouldn't be spayed while in heat, but we've no choice in Sheba's case. She's always in heat."

The Rousseaus left Sheba to be spayed. The cat would remain

with us as a boarder for three weeks while they were vacationing in Canada.

I performed the surgery just before dinner. She seemed to be coming out of it normally, and when I checked her again before going to bed, she was shivering as animals do when they start to awaken from anesthesia. The corneal reflex of her eye was strong and I went to bed with Sheba easy on my mind.

After breakfast, I checked all the surgical cases of the day before. That built-in panic button of alarm went off the moment I looked into Sheba's cage. She was stiff and motionless and her blue eyes were open wide, staring at me, yet unseeing. I quickly opened the door and felt her chest.

Lub-dub, lub-dub—nothing.

Had I heard it? Was it a heartbeat I had heard or had I felt the beat of my own pulse in my thumb? I reached for a nearby stethoscope. All was quiet now. I could not hear a thing.

But it must have been the heart! I told myself. It must have been! In desperation, I roughly massaged Sheba's heart through her rib cage and anxiously felt again.

Lub-dub!

It had been the heart I had heard! I quickly massaged some more, hoping that the heart would not stop beating again. I pushed her rib cage in and then let it spring out and then massaged some more.

Massage and feel. There was a tremulous beat.

Massage and feel. *Lub-dub.* A long pause, and my heart stopped too. But then once again, *lub-dub.*

Massage and feel—*lub-dub, lub-dub*—and finally there was a stronger, more rhythmical *lub-dub, lub-dub, lub-dub.*

I breathed a slow and cautious sigh. At least the heart was started again, but the cat was not breathing. I gave her mouth-to-mouth resuscitation and watched her lungs fill with my own breath. In then out, in then out, but Sheba did not start breathing.

The cat was cold and quite stiff. I ran with her into the kitchen, where it was warmer, and called to Mame to bring some of Marilyn's doll blankets. I worked over that cat for more than twenty-five minutes. The heartbeat was strong now, and as long as the cat had a heartbeat, I would not give her up. I kept breathing for her and tears of frustration and despair were beginning to form. I blinked very rapidly so my tears flowed through my lachrymal ducts down into my nose. I can still remember how I had to keep sniffing to keep my nose from running.

At last it came, that magical, wonderful moment—that first hesitant quiver—that first uncertain breath.

I waited, but she did not take another breath, so I pressed on her rib cage and let the ribs spring back into position. There it was—the second breath.

I waited a moment now and did not touch her, hoping the carbon dioxide buildup would trigger the breathing center of her brain. Finally she started. She took one breath, then another, and finally yet another. It was like pulling teeth, bringing that cat back to life.

"Mame!" I called. "Please light the oven and set it at the lowest possible temperature. And you know that large blue-and-white ovenproof platter in the cupboard? Will you bring it here?"

I covered the platter with several layers of aluminum foil and then put one of the doll blankets over the foil. I placed the cat on the blanket and tucked Sheba in the oven, leaving the door open. All I could think of were the owner's words: "We think the world of her. . . . She acts more like a dog than a cat. . . . She'll fetch things when you throw them for her. . . . She's a regular clown. . . . She even sits and watches TV with us."

They had good reason to love their cat. In addition to being an interesting and intelligent pet, Sheba was one of the most beautiful Sealpoint Siamese cats I had ever seen.

"She's just so cold, Mame. Her body temperature is so low that she's no longer capable of warming up by herself. She must have some external source of heat."

I checked Sheba's temperature: 92 degrees, a good nine degrees below normal! We continued to watch Sheba like two hawks, and every fifteen minutes either Mame or I would turn the cat over on her other side and massage her in an effort to stimulate her circulation. We'd rub her cold feet and tail and ears. We repeatedly wet her corneas with ophthalmic solution to prevent her eyes from drying out.

Finally, over two hours later, Sheba was breathing smoothly and her heart sounds were normal. Her temperature had reached 96 degrees.

I left the rest of the nursing up to Mame.

"Keep turning her, Mame. She has no eye reflexes yet and her lids keep falling open, so be sure to keep putting these drops in—they're like artificial tears."

I started giving fluids intravenously, letting them drip slowly from a bottle I had warmed in a dishpan of warm water. The cat was cold enough, I figured; no sense in making matters harder for the poor animal by dripping cold fluids into her.

I finished treating hospital cases with John, checking on Sheba at frequent intervals. Just before afternoon office hours, I took the cat's temperature again. It was almost 100 degrees, so I turned the oven off and wrapped her gently in the doll blankets. I tapped one eyeball gently; there was a faint incipient wink. Her eye reflex was beginning to return.

"Mother! What will Daddy say about your sticking a cat in the oven!" Marilyn, just home from school, had been surprised to see Mame tending the cat, bent over the open oven door. "Can I wet the cat's eyes and take care of it for you, Mother?" Marilyn begged. "I asked Mame and she told me to come ask you."

"Why, yes, Marilyn. Mame and I would appreciate some help."

I had no qualms about entrusting the cat, at this point, to Marilyn. If Marilyn once promised to do something, she'd do it, and I knew that if anything changed at all, she could be depended on to come and tell me.

Marilyn set up a doll's table, covered it with a clean white towel and placed the ophthalmoscope, the thermometer in a jar of alcohol, cotton and a stack of towels carefully on top as if it were a treatment table. Marilyn was in her element; she was happy because she was helping something.

Raymond took over the tedious vigil after dinner. By this time, Sheba could raise her head and blink her eyes. Ray carried a portable kennel for me from the storeroom and placed it in the room just off the kitchen that Joe used for his photographic work. It was a warm room and very accessible, so that I could easily continue to monitor the cat throughout the night.

Since Sheba could blink her eyes now, I switched to an eye ointment instead of the drops. Ray transferred the cat to her new quarters, wrapping the doll blankets around her. I continued to give her fluids, and when I went to bed I set the alarm so that it would awaken me in one hour. I did not turn the house thermostat down. All through the night, I got up and checked on Sheba to make sure she continued to improve. I wanted no stomach-turning surprise that morning.

We kept Sheba in our home all the next day, and again that night, before I finally felt it was safe to return her to the main kennel room.

Mame thought it was all a miracle. She was never so right. "No pulse, no breathing, no heartbeat, temperature ice cold and stiff as a board—that cat was dead and didn't know it!" Mame told the rest of the family at breakfast. "That cat would not be alive today if it was not for your wife," she said to Joe as she placed the coffeepot in front of him.

"It wouldn't be alive right now if it weren't for you, Mame!" I said as I mopped up my egg yolk with a piece of toast. "You're the one who kept her going all day by turning her, massaging her and putting the drops in her eyes." I took a sip of coffee. "In fact," I added, "Sheba wouldn't be alive now if it weren't for Marilyn and Ray too. We all worked very hard."

I was honestly proud and pleased with all our efforts. Sheba had been ripped from the jaws of death, so to speak, back from the netherworld.

I was feeling pretty pleased with myself all morning until, treating hospital cases, I came to Sheba.

I felt sick. There was Sheba before me, heartbeat fine and strong, and breathing regular—but that was all!

Sheba had become a vegetable.

She was blind, she was deaf, and she was dumb. She had no sense of balance, could not walk, had no sense of smell and no sense of touch.

I was mortified.

Was I going to return this creature to its loving owners as a zombie? A feline zombie?

It would have been better if she had remained dead. . . .

I sighed and petted Sheba. I flicked her magnificent whiskers gently with my index finger, but they did not twitch; Sheba could not feel me.

I picked her up, her body unresisting, and I sat with her in my lap.

"John!" I called. "Bring me a small amount of canned tuna, will you?"

I held a blob of it in my hand right under the cat's nose. No response; she could not smell the food.

I decided to try something.

I took a tiny portion, about the size of a bean, and prying Sheba's mouth open, I pushed the food inside toward the base of her tongue. Then I closed her mouth.

Gulp!

Sheba swallowed it!

"The swallow reflex is still there, John!" I called excitedly. "She can swallow food if it's put into her mouth!"

The next day Sheba managed to get up by herself, but she lost her balance, and fell repeatedly. She kept trying, though, and eventually she could stand and keep her balance. When she tried her first step, she collapsed, but Sheba was one smart cat. Having fallen against the wall of the kennel, when she got up to try again she deliberately leaned against the kennel wall for support and kept on trying to walk. I attempted to imagine how the animal must feel. Everything was as black as night to her, she was in strange surroundings, there were no sounds to guide her, no smells. . . .

Sheba paced the kennel wall to wall, hugging the sides for support. That was all there was at first—that primitive urge to keep herself moving. It was nature's way, I suppose, the best way to get the circulation going again in order to carry the necessary nutrients to the tissues—vital supplies to keep the tissues alive and help them regain their functions.

The next day Sheba could walk unsupported, but being blind, she'd bump into the opposite wall of the kennel, so now she depended on the four walls of her cage as a guide rather than a support. Around and around she would go. One-two-three-four, one-two-three-four. If it had been a circular kennel, I would have become dizzy watching her.

Her sense of touch returned next, as evidenced by the twitching of her whiskers when they contacted anything.

Next, the olfactory sense came back. When we put a dish of food in her cage, she walked diagonally across the kennel floor, guided by her sense of smell.

The next day there was sweet music. Sheba meowed! It was the first sound she had made since I had anesthetized her.

On the sixth day, Sheba started grooming herself—always a welcome sight with a sick animal.

Sheba was still deaf and blind, however, and I worried about her. How could one make all this comprehensible to a client?

Apprehensively, I checked the calendar. The Rousseaus were due to return in two weeks and I was afraid that the circulation to some of Sheba's vital areas had been inadequate for so long as to have caused irreparable damage to certain tissues. I feared that the auditory and optic nerves had been damaged beyond nature's power to repair them; most likely I was going to send the Rousseaus home with a deaf and blind cat.

What more could I do? I fed her well and gave her vitamin and mineral supplements. I brushed her and groomed her and played that maddening waiting game. . . .

Marilyn kept up Sheba's morale. From the moment she returned home from school each day, she lavished attention on the cat, and I truly believe that in some intangible way, the love Sheba received from my Marilyn really helped her recovery.

On the ninth day, I found Sheba curled in her kennel, sleeping peacefully.

"Pss-pst! Pss-wss-wss." I pss-wssed at her and her ears twitched! Sheba awakened and turned her head toward my sounds!

Oh, what a flood of encouragement I felt! If the auditory nerves were not permanently damaged, I dared to hope now that in time the ocular nerves would function again too.

Two days later the last miracle came to pass and Sheba could see. Our hours of keeping her corneas moist had paid off, for there had been no drying and consequent sloughing of opaque dead corneal tissue. Now, with sight restored, Sheba looked directly at me through bright and shining heavenly blue eyes.

The next day the phone rang.

"Dr. Logue? It's Mrs. Rousseau. We're back early. Would it be convenient to call for Sheba this afternoon? How is she, anyway?"

"She's fine, Mrs. Rousseau. Yes, this afternoon would be fine."

Sheba was obviously happy to see her owners, and responded especially to Mr. Rousseau.

"This is the most remarkable cat, Dr. Logue," effused Mrs. Rousseau. "It's my husband's cat really—I've never seen him take to an animal so before." Mrs. Rousseau was smiling and animated, and without waiting to take a breath, she continued: "Sheba looks just wonderful. I can see she was well cared for. Thank you, Dr. Logue. Thank you very much."

"There is something you must know," I began to tell them. "I almost lost Sheba. I don't know what went wrong, but she almost died before she finally recovered from anesthesia. It was terrible—"

"Oh, now, you were probably overly concerned. That's why we always bring our pets here—because we both feel you're so interested and very conscientious. You have such a way with animals."

"But actually, Mrs. Rousseau, that cat had a terrible time and we really almost lost her. Sheba had no pulse, even her breathing stopped and her heart—"

"Why, how frightful!" Mrs. Rousseau interrupted. "I'm so glad we were on vacation and remained dumb and happy, so to speak." And she took a second look at Sheba, who was purring and rubbing her cheek and ear against Mrs. Rousseau's handbag. "Well," she continued, "it's quite obvious she's just fine now," and with a bright smile, Mrs. Rousseau seemed to dismiss it all. "We knew Sheba would be all right if we left her with you." And they were gone.

I somehow felt let down. All those day-by-day little miracles, and they never gave me a chance to describe any of them!

I am not formally religious, but I felt somehow, for a moment, that what some people would call God had just been taken for granted.

About a week later, Mrs. Rousseau phoned. Sheba was fine, she reported, was eating well, and was her calm old self again. She showed no signs of being in heat and all was peace and quiet. The male toms had given up and gone home. There was just one thing that puzzled her.

"What is that, Mrs. Rousseau?" I asked.

"Well, I don't know how to say it, but—was Sheba's tail ever injured, to your knowledge? Caught in the kennel door or something?"

"Absolutely not, Mrs. Rousseau, and I know that John would have told me if he accidentally caught the tail while feeding her or cleaning her kennel. As I tried to tell you, we had a stormy time with Sheba and all of us worked very tirelessly over her. No—I'm sure I would have been told if her tail had been injured. How does it look to you?"

"Well, toward the end there is a warm, hottish swelling and the tip behind this feels thin and stiff."

Gangrene! "Bring her right over—now—Mrs. Rousseau! I must see her!"

Sheba did have gangrene of her tail.

This time Mrs. Rousseau listened to me.

"Her circulation was at such a low ebb for a while that the very end tissues in the tip of her tail lost their supply of blood and died. The only thing I can do now to save Sheba is to amputate her tail above the gangrenous area."

I dreaded reanesthetizing this cat, considering what had happened the last time. I used short-acting sodium pentothal and by the time I was securing the last bit of tape on the bandage, she was swishing her tipless tail and groggily weaving her head.

The Queen of Sheba was going to be just fine. Everything had been restored to life but the tip of her tail!

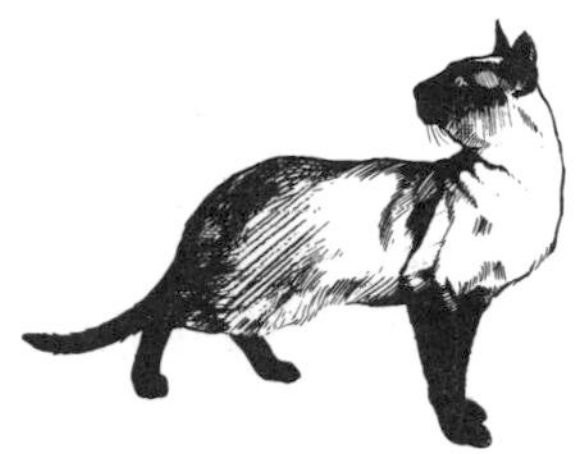

19

"Be sure to mark Saturday the twenty-first on the calendar," Joe said at the dinner table one evening. He tapped the ash buildup from his cigar and continued: "We're having a farewell dinner party in honor of Ron Hall. He's had a promotion and is being transferred to the West Coast. It's important that we both be there."

Naturally, the phone shrilled like some nagging termagant just as I was getting dressed for Ron Hall's dinner. I looked at Joe out of the corner of my eye and I could see that look settling on his face, but he didn't say anything. I let the phone scold me twice more before I picked up the receiver—to be greeted by a real live termagant.

"But can't you possibly call another veterinarian this time, Miss Grayson? Matters are such here that it would be most difficult to get out to you." I hated to ask her to phone someone else, for I was her regular vet. Miss Grayson had no way of knowing how much Joe had been counting on this evening.

"No. I really can't. You know all my animals. You're my regular vet and I'm so worried about this mare. I tried to save you a trip by doctoring her myself. I knew she was in labor, so I gave her some pituitary extract to help speed things along. She really strained after I gave her the shot, but then suddenly all labor stopped. It was the oddest thing! Now she looks strange to me. I never saw her sweat so before, and she's starting to hang her head. I'm becoming very concerned—"

"Say no more." I interrupted her to save time. "I'll drop everything and drive right over." My scalp prickled all around my hairline just at the thought of what might be the mare's problem. "If the trouble is what I think it is, Miss Grayson, you should prepare yourself for a bit of bad news."

I turned toward Joe. He knotted his tie impatiently, then tightened it viciously with a last jerk of his hands.

"I'm sorry, Joe—I really tried."

"Forget it, Jeanne. Just forget the whole evening." His tone was coldly polite, but I knew the depth of his anger by the way his eyes changed color. In silence, I tucked the small red rim of his tie up under the back of his shirt collar so that it didn't show.

During the drive to Miss Grayson's, my stomach felt upset and I kept burping up bitter, bilious-tasting fluid. No matter what choice I had made—the dinner or Miss Grayson—I would still have heartburn, I supposed, because there was no completely right choice for me in this instance; I would be wrong either way.

I wondered whatever had possessed Miss Grayson to give Pitocin and where she ever gained possession of the stuff. My client had a number of horses north of Woodstock, loved her animals, but also loved her role as one of the "horsy set." A shirt and scarf, jodhpurs and riding boots—this was Miss Grayson's uniform. She took great pride in her knowledge of horses and was very critical of my work. This was nothing personal. It was her nature to be critical with everybody, for she was a self-appointed authority on many subjects. Medicine, horticulture, gourmet cooking, real estate—you name it. Miss Grayson was an authority.

"Just when did you give this Pitocin injection, Miss Grayson, and how soon after it did you say she stopped straining?" I was washing my arm as she answered.

"About one half hour before I called you. She gave two tremendous pushes and then bang! She stopped. She just stood very still and then she started sweating."

"How long had she been in labor before you injected her?"

"Oh, she had just started, so I gave her the injection to hurry her along. I know a good bit about these things." She spoke as though teaching me something. "There's an obstetrician I know who induces labor in the women. He never sits up all night to deliver someone's baby. He plans all his deliveries. . . ." And she prattled on—the authority—about how she too helped nature along. She didn't mean to honk her own horn, but she believed that she gave a pretty good needle; the horse hardly flinched when it went in.

By this time I had donned a shoulder-length glove and inserted my arm very gently into the mare's vagina. The cervix was not dilated, so I withdrew my arm and inserted it carefully into her rectum. I did not have far to reach.

I felt a sharp little hoof and part of a leg, which was protruding into the rectum. There was an enormous tear in the rectal wall and the rent in the uterus at the site of the rupture was like a gaping tent flap. Placental fluids and blood had poured into the peritoneal cavity and feces had fallen down and had dropped into the uterus.

"Oh, Miss Grayson!" I wailed. "Little do you know the mischief and the damage you've done!"

"What do you mean?"

"Your injection. You helped nature along, all right! You brought on powerful contractions prematurely. That mare's insides are like a bomb went off in there—everything's torn asunder! "

"But that's impossible! Just impossible!"

I shook my head in despair.

"Before *any* veterinarian injects *any* Pitocin into *any* laboring animal, a vaginal exam first and perhaps also a rectal exam is a *must.* One must make sure the cervix is dilated and the fetus is in the proper position. If Pitocin is given while the cervix is still firm, and not dilated, the uterus may rupture when the strong contractions begin. You get a good, strong, healthy mare like this bearing down powerfully from a good stiff dose of Pitocin before her cervix is dilated, and she's bearing down on a closed system! Where's the foal to go? Through the thin, stretched uterine wall, that's where!"

"I don't believe it! That's impossible!" she repeated. Her face was ashen. "I've seen you give that injection a number of times."

"Sure I have, but I've always made sure that the cervix was open first, and that the foal was in the right position. Well?" I looked in despair at the miserable animal and then at Miss Grayson again. "Do you want to try to save the mare's life? We still may have a very slim chance, but she'll never foal again. I really believe it's best to put her down."

"Ridiculous! This is all impossible!"

Miss Grayson could not accept the fact that she had just about killed her mare. I suggested that she either euthanize the poor beast or let me try to remove the foal and repair the damage as best I could. I did not spare her feelings when I described what a gory job that would be, for it would involve an embryotomy—the use of obstetrical chains and sawing up the foal inside the mother until I obtained pieces small enough to remove bit by bit through the hole in the rectum. My third suggestion, if the first two were unacceptable, was to call another veterinarian for a second opinion.

Miss Grayson accepted my third suggestion.

I heard from a client the following week that the mare had dropped dead that next morning and that the foul, shredded mess inside her was discovered after she was sold, when she was being cut up for dog food. Folks claim Miss Grayson never quite got over what she had done, and I must say I can understand why. It was a bitter lesson she had received. Miss Grayson, the self-appointed authority on so many things, so wise in her own conceit, had paid an exorbitant tuition fee for her education.

I returned home from Miss Grayson's depressed. Dead and dying animals always do this to me. I showered and dressed again and drove alone to meet Joe at the dinner party. The dinner was over, of course, by the time I arrived, but I found Joe and sat down in a vacant chair next to him just as after-dinner speeches were ending. I was embarrassed by my lateness, but at least, I thought to alleviate my guilt, at least I was putting in an appearance. I was tired and discouraged and the dead foal and doomed mare had me in a low mood. I would rather have stayed home.

We socialized a bit after the speeches and John Murray, sitting at our table, who knew Joe and also knew my line of work, told me of an amusing conversation that had taken place during dinner.

"All the men and their wives were here except you, Jeanne. You were the only one missing." I cringed. "One of the four couples at the table were strangers, and seeing your empty place setting, asked Joe where his wife was. Joe, here, didn't crack a smile, but in a very matter-of-fact voice said that you were sitting up with a sick horse! The couple started laughing, thinking Joe was trying to be funny. The rest of us started laughing because we all knew that what he said was probably true."

"And I started laughing," Joe joined the conversation, "because I found it amusing to realize that everyone was laughing about a different thing!"

The affair came to an end and there was a long drive home—alone, because we had come in separate cars.

Joe was still unhappy about my attending the mare and being so late for dinner. Yes, he could understand that I had to go. . . .

"Oh, hell, Jeanne. I don't know what the answer is."

I had noticed the subtle change in Joe's attitude lately. He was beginning to leave for work with a detectable air of detachment rather than with his usual warm goodbye, and he was quieter and less communicative. He seemed to brood rather than to concentrate on things anymore. I thought I understood what was wrong, but I asked Joe nevertheless. Might as well flop it on the table, as Joe always said.

Once asked, he laid his thoughts straight on the line and thrashed them out as one would musty draperies and dusty throw rugs that had been mildewing in some neglected house for a long time.

"The very thought of continuing year after year with never a free weekend, evening, or even an uninterrupted meal—to look forward to that type of hectic schedule is intolerable to me.

"The idea of hiring another veterinarian is not a bit encouraging—what luck have you had so far? Sure, I know you've tried and it's not your fault—but what's to change? We could go on for a couple of years before you find someone you think is suitable as an assistant or a partner. I've lost patience with waiting.

"I'm sick and tired of receiving Christmas cards addressed to Dr. and Mr. Logue, and when Mr. Hoffman, the gardener, comes, he always asks for *you!* 'What jobs does Dr. Logue want done?' right to my face, as though I were some goddamn lackey or something. I'm beginning to feel like a toady in my own home, for Christ's sake!

"There are two children who need you, who demand and

deserve your attention, and you want *another* baby? Jesus, you're so stupid!" He snorted derisively and paced the bedroom floor.

He went on and on, without the slightest hesitation, listing his discontents. They were many, all valid, and I listened, not suprised by what he said, but subdued by his barrage because it was more intense and splenetic than I had expected.

There was a stony silence and a tangible wall of tension as we went to bed, and stiffly, back to back, we both lay in the darkness, unhappy.

At two thirty-five in the morning, the phone rang and I had to leave to tend to a cow with a prolapsed uterus. It was on the farm next to Stemmler's, and on the way home I stopped at my special quiet spot. I had frequented this lake on several occasions when I felt the need of a bit of solitary contemplation. Tonight, Orion was reflected in the lake again, and there being something about this particular constellation from which I could gain strength and regain my equanimity, I studied his stars for a while in an effort to center down, query myself and perhaps organize my harassed emotions and troubled thoughts.

This night, Joe and I had had our first serious altercation in all our married years and it upset me terribly. My cheeks were still flaming and my heart still pounded like a sledge hammer against my chest. I felt disoriented and shaky inside. I pondered long and hard on what had been over the years, what there was now, and what might be in the future.

The years so far had been pure gold and full of happiness. In the early days, Joe had been very enthusiastic about my being a veterinarian. Before we were married, he had known of my desire to practice, so he did not enter into our relationship blind. He knew the way of life in store for us—but did he *really* know? At that time how could he possibly have known what it would really be like?

I recalled Joe's sales pitch during our courting days. He wanted a professional woman as his wife. The two professions, medicine and engineering, would complement each other, he said persuasively, and then he would tell me how he planned to design and build me a portable x-ray machine. In fact, in the early years of our marriage, Joe did build me a fine instrument cabinet, with sliding glass doors. He constructed a beautiful large oak desk too, with drawers that didn't stick, and the finish he put on that oak was like satin. I remembered how pleased I was and how proud. The furniture was more than the result of good carpentry; Joe's work reflected the pride and the skill of a cabinetmaker, but then, everything he did was done to perfection.

Yes, he certainly had been supportive in the early days, and I supposed now a little wistfully, as I stared at the lake, that the novelty of having a busy veterinarian as a wife was beginning to wear a bit thin.

I turned my mind to the present. I reevaluated all the complaints Joe had hurled at me at bedtime and I tried very hard, with both love and understanding, to see his point of view. I took a hard critical look at myself to determine how well or how poorly I measured up to his needs, and, for the first time in my life, I began to feel a bit uncertain about myself.

Of one thing, however, I was still certain. One thing was firm, it was absolute and it was enduring. It was also very simple: I loved the man with all my being.

"What about the future?" I queried myself aloud in the darkness. And then I reasoned to myself. "We both have too many good years tucked under our belts to risk losing now. We have the best family in the world and we all get along with each other so well. There are just too many good times invested and too many future dividends to be gained. It is not worth risking.

"There must be some way," I determined. I clenched my

jaws stubbornly and closed my eyes. "There must be some way to be happy and have both—the family and the profession. Greedy I may be, but there's got to be a way. Somewhere, some way, a door will surely open." I opened my eyes.

High in the sky he was as I looked up at Orion, resolute and strong against the blackness. I had made up my mind.

I closed my mental ledger book and started to drive home. As is so often the way, I felt better for no other reason than that a decision had been made.

When I arrived home, I went directly to the office. I sat down at my desk and with an unwavering hand, I started writing an ad for the AVMA journal which began: "Large and Small Animal Practice for Sale. . . ."

I agreed with all the items on Joe's bill of particulars except one. There was one item about which Joe was wrong—dead wrong.

I was not stupid and I wished he hadn't said that to me.

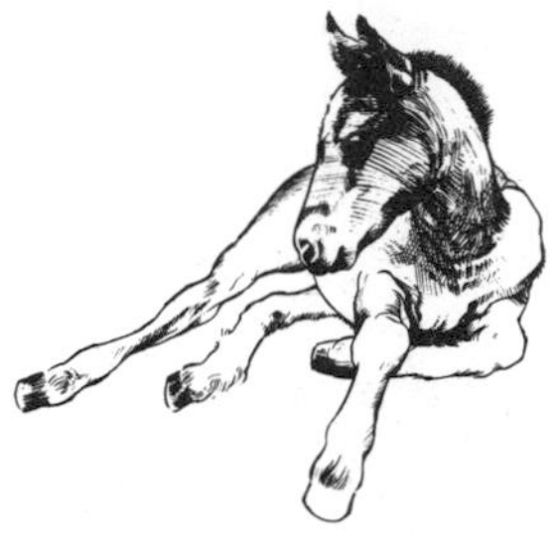

20

While I hadn't been successful in finding a suitable veterinarian to hire as an assistant, to Joe's pleasure and my surprise I had immediate success when it came to selling the practice. I never dreamed it would happen so fast. We had just about two months left to find a place to live, while the new doctor gave the vet he was working for ample notice and made financial arrangements with the bank. I felt rather sorry for the veterinarian who had to find a replacement in two months.

My last large-animal call came from Mr. Bemis, and I was glad I was still in town so that I could attend. There were seven members in the Bemis family. The mister and missis, Cissy, Benjie, Roy, Bert and Blue Bell. Blue Bell was the horse, and I have seen fewer animals so loved and so much a part of a family as that horse. The Bemises had two homes. One was a farm about five miles outside of town, where they lived each spring and summer; the second, a house in town, was their winter quarters. Blue Bell made the trip each spring and fall with the family and she was always as happy as the children to get out in the country again.

Kingston and the surrounding areas had a special charm to me in those days. There were rows of houses and even sidewalks, but out back behind a house, more often than not, was a shed of sorts which sheltered a horse or two. There were a good number of saddle horses in Kingston twenty years ago; the Sunday-afternoon drive there took the form of the Sunday-afternoon ride. I loved it. Because of the liberal zoning laws, Blue Bell was a welcome member in town during the late-fall and winter months.

I remembered the first time the Bemises called me to examine Blue Bell. It was on a May morning about a year before, and the air was sweet and fresh. I passed by sunny patches of yellow coltsfoot and saw the fiddlehead ferns starting to unfurl. I was filled with my usual springtime exhilaration. How could I help but be joyful? A happy heart is good medicine and I prescribed freely for myself. A community of May apples, or mandrakes, waved their parasols at me as I drove along. I knew that if I stopped and lifted one of the umbrellalike leaves, I'd find the single white flower hiding beneath, close to the stalk, shy and fragile. Mandrakes were sociable plants, I figured, for they always grew in small groves in close company.

Apple trees were in bloom everywhere, and as I pulled into the Bemises' barnyard, the air was heavy with the scent of lilacs. Blue Bell was down when I saw her and could not rise. She was lying in her roomy stall, which had one window. She was on her side, with her back slightly arched, well bedded with deep pilings of sweet-smelling straw.

At the sight of me, Mrs. Bemis and her oldest child, Cissy, started crying. Mr. Bemis very politely and almost apologetically explained why I had been called.

"We ain't doubting Doc Ferris's word, you understand. We think the world of him and have had him for years—but hang it all, we just love Blue Bell so much." He looked away from me and I heard him sniff. "Doc Ferris says to put the horse down, that Blue Bell is hopeless, but we just can't bring ourselves to do it. We feel we just had to have another opinion before we did anything so final. No offense to Doc Ferris, mind you." Then he added respectfully, "Would you take a look at her and see what you think?"

Mrs. Bemis sat herself down on a bale of hay, her face like that of the mother of a condemned child, waiting for the sentence. The rest of her children, like chicks, gathered around her.

Mr. Bemis lay down beside the horse's head and talked to Blue Bell. I've seldom heard a man's voice so soft and gentle, and it seemed incongruous to me at first, coming from such a big, strong mountain of a man. Mr. Bemis must have been about six feet four and that's what he reminded me of—one of our strapping grizzly-bear mountain men of a bygone era.

I knew the horse had pain in the lumbar area and I tried to be as gentle as I could. I examined her rectally and could feel the uterus and ovaries through the rectal wall. Next, I was able to touch her left kidney. Blue Bell shuddered and quivered with a sudden stab of pain and gave a low moan. Her kidney was large and lobulated and I could feel a distinct firm mass which involved the distal end. I told them that I believed the horse had a tumor involving her kidney. This explained the back pain, the gradual loss in weight, the unthriftiness, and the occasional bloody urine they had seen Blue Bell pass from time to time.

"Doc Ferris thought she had nephritis and that we ought to put her down."

"He was probably right about the nephritis, but I'm afraid there is also a growth involved."

Mrs. Bemis started crying all the harder. Her husband looked at her in anguish and then turned and said, "I just can't do it—not today. Isn't there anything you can think of to try? Anything at all for the pain?"

I told them that Dr. Ferris's suggestion was probably right and certainly humane, and while there was no cure, I would do what I could to ease the horse's condition and make her more comfortable until they could bring themselves to decide what to do.

Blue Bell was no longer eating or drinking and I suspected her spirits were being broken by the pain and anxiety and fear. I gave her what supportive treatment I could. I fed her intravenously, pumped in electrolytes and vitamins and dosed her with antibiotics. I had read recently that cortisone was found to help in stress conditions and that there sometimes was a remission in certain tumors when this drug was used. I administered two grams of cortisone. I wasn't sure how much good it would do, but at least it would act as an anti-inflammatory, and for this alone it was worth a try. If the swelling in her kidneys went down, it would relieve the pain. I obtained a urine specimen and helped them rig a sling to support the horse in an upright condition.

Nobody was very encouraged; we all knew we were buying time. There were sad and anxious faces all about and no one noticed the lilacs or the nodding purple panicles of the giant wisteria tree that clambered up one side of the barn and onto the roof. People kept gathering all during the time I was there. I never saw such a congregation. There were children of assorted ages, but most of them were teen-agers; it was Saturday, and with no school to attend, they came to the Bemises' to watch Blue Bell in somber silence. Some of their mothers and fathers were there too, and even a few grandfathers. Everyone kept looking toward one man in particular. He was in his nineties and I was told later that Mr. Purdy was the great-grandfather of young Bert Bemis's best friend, Fred, who lived on the next farm. Mr. Purdy was very lean, had prominent cheekbones and alert bright eyes that were set deep in their sockets. He had been a genuine cowboy out West in his day and was looked upon by all, myself included—for I must say he had a certain charisma—as the cow and horse expert. He wore a wide-brimmed cowboy hat that he let hang loosely down his back, the tie secured around his throat. He also had on a cowboy shirt, and a lanyard around his neck. This was held together by a ring of bone carved into the shape of a steer's head with graceful long horns extending to either side.

"She ain't agoing to be getting up again, Cissy girl," he predicted, laying a kind hand on the girl's shining hair. "I've seen many a horse in my day and I know. I can tell. You'll just have to be brave and face up to it, Cissy. Blue Bell will never leave her stall alive."

I learned later that all the teen-agers present used to be the toddlers that Blue Bell would patiently ride around on her back, two and three at a time. The horse and these children had remained friends over the years, and the youngsters, growing up now, had come in Blue Bell's hour of peril.

The phone awakened me at a quarter to seven the next morning. The excited voice of Mr. Bemis came over the wire.

"Oh, lord, Doc. I went to the barn first thing this morning to look in on Blue Bell, and as I entered, she whinnied at me. And, Doc—oh, lord, what a beautiful sight!" I thought he was going to cry. "Blue Bell was supporting her own weight. Yes, sir! Standing on her own four feet, she was! She even drank some water from her bucket. Oh, lord! Thanks, Doc. You did a wonderful job. Wait till I tell Jim Purdy—he'll never believe it."

Tumor cells had washed down with the formation of urine, and a urinalysis by a friend of mine in charge of the local hospital's tumor clinic confirmed my suspicions. Blue Bell had a carcinoma. We discussed the cortisone therapy, and while it was his experience that malignant lymphomas seemed to respond best, he felt it would be foolish to discontinue using cortisone in view of the marked improvement of the patient.

I felt very much like the Brave Little Tailor in the fairy

tale—the one who wore a belt in which the words "Seven in One Blow" had been woven. With Blue Bell and me it was a matter of "Seven in one shot," for in helping this animal, with one injection of cortisone, I made the entire family happy. It was a good feeling, believe me. Dr. Ferris was delighted with Blue Bell's improvement, and while everybody knew that the horse's days were numbered, she would be able to get about and be free from pain at least for a while. It was with a certain amount of happy excitement that I continued to medicate Blue Bell, gradually reducing the dosage of the cortisone. She started eating and even put on a little weight. Jim Purdy claimed that now he had seen everything and his blue eyes flashed with pleasure.

"I never would have believed that a horse with such a backache as Blue Bell had would ever git up again. Bad sign, such a backache in a horse—bad sign," the old man claimed.

News of Blue Bell's backache cure must have spread, for one day a stranger came to the office without an animal. He waited his turn and after three dogs and one cat, he arose stiffly from his chair and came into the examining room. He presented his problem. The patient was—himself. It seems he was suffering from a bad back—in fact, his back had been "killing him" for almost six months. He claimed he had been to all kinds of doctors, but that they all "didn't do no good." Having been told about Blue Bell by Jim Purdy, he had made a trip to the Bemises' farm to witness the miraculous cure and had made up his mind.

"Old Jim Purdy is your greatest fan, young lady. He swears by you," Mr. Sewell said as he gingerly massaged the small of his back and shifted from left to right to left foot again in an effort to ease his discomfort. "And the Bemises!" He continued to shift in a swaying motion from side to side. "Why, they'd let you take care of their kids anytime—so I was wondering and hoping maybe you could do something for my back."

Mr. Sewell was not joking or pulling my leg at all. He was serious! Absolutely serious!

I told him with effusive apologies that much as I would like to help him, I couldn't. Legally, I couldn't so much as prescribe an aspirin. (My fingers just itched, though, to give *him* a dose of cortisone to see what would happen.)

"My license to practice medicine is legal for all animals *except* the human, Mr. Sewell. It would be against the law to prescribe for you. I'm afraid you will simply have to try another M.D."

At dinner, I told the family about Mr. Sewell's unusual request.

"I felt sorry for the poor man. He really looked to be in misery, but can you imagine anyone actually coming to me, a veterinarian, for treatment?" I was grinning from ear to ear because of the novelty and odd humor of it all.

"Well, I wouldn't mind your doctoring me, Ma. I don't blame that man for coming," Ray said loyally, and I will admit that I was touched, for there was a sincere ring of pride in his voice.

"Hell, I wouldn't let your mother near any of you," Joe boomed, with a twinkle in his eyes. They were a lighter shade of brown now and I knew he was teasing. "After your mother jabbed a needle into my thumb late one night when I was helping her sew up a dog that had been swiped by a bear, I wouldn't let her near me with a Band-Aid!" We all laughed and Joe tousled my hair jokingly.

The dog Joe had been helping me with had very tough skin and the tears in it were extensive and ragged. I trimmed the wound edges and Joe was trying to hold the skin together while I did the sewing.

"Mind you, watch that needle as it comes through the skin," he had warned, squinting a bit as the smoke arose from his perennial cigar, which was clenched between his teeth. I was making abrupt stabs with the needle against the tough, elastic skin in order to get the needle through.

"N'yah, you haven't a thing to worry about."

Pop!

The needle suddenly pierced the tough skin, smack into the fleshy part of Joe's thumb! The air became blue as he shook his thumb and then held it out to examine it.

"Christ—now you've done it! All I need is to come down with hepatitis or distemper."

"You already have the latter! Ha! Ha!" Oh, how I laughed. The harder I laughed, the madder he became. . . .

But all this about Joe's thumb, Mr. Sewell and my first trip to the Bemis farm was all history now. The thing I would always remember was that Blue Bell and the Bemis clan had one extra happy year together. All the past summer Blue Bell had roamed free and followed the various members of the family around like a dog. She was truly a family pet, and if she wasn't with this person or another, Mrs. Bemis could always find Blue Bell under her favorite apple tree in the yard, daydreaming or napping while standing, lulled by the hum of the flies and the honeybees busy in the clover. She had enjoyed the whole summer this way, spending her days in peace and contentment. In the fall, as usual, they had moved back to town, and the winter had passed and the spring had arrived once more. I was on my way, glad we had not moved yet and that I was still in town, for Blue Bell's time had finally come. Blue Bell was dying.

The Bemises were determined to get Blue Bell back to the farm once more, to die in happy surroundings. I was asked to come along so that if there was an accident while she was being moved and Blue Bell broke a leg or something, I would be immediately available to inject a barbiturate and put her out of her misery.

I have seen many kindnesses to animals, I have seen acts

of great love, I have seen many a person cater to and pamper the little ones—the toy breeds like the Pekingese and the toy poodle—Mrs. Wilson and Mimi immediately come to my mind—but oddly enough, it was the Bemises who topped them all with their huge old mare.

I parked the car and walked down the driveway to the shed behind their house, passing clumps of yellow daffodils and blue violets which were blooming helter-skelter in profusion.

The Bemises had taken a mattress from one of their double beds and somehow, with the aid of the men in the neighborhood, they had managed to get it under Blue Bell. Under the mattress, for rigidity, they had wrestled into position a heavy four-by-eight-foot piece of plywood.

The Bemises had many friends and fortunately, as it turned out for Blue Bell, many of them were in the construction business. I will never forget the man operating the fork-lift. To make the patient accessible, while causing her the least discomfort, Mr. Bemis knocked down one whole wall of Blue Bell's shed. The fork-lift operator, whose name was Angelo, was a short, stocky fellow with a cauliflower nose that suggested he might have been a prizefighter at one time. He wore a black cap with a visor that could be turned up out of the way and snapped to the front of the cap. Angelo wore the visor down as a sunshade, and while he worked, I could see the metal snap glint in the dark material whenever the sun's rays hit it. He also wore what looked like a blacksmith's apron. It was made of black leather, and had a row of large pockets sewn around the front hem.

Angelo managed the fork-lift with great skill and deftly lifted the plywood, the mattress and Blue Bell while the rest of the men steadied the free end of the horse's bed so it would not tip and fall off the fork. They all walked along with the fork-lift, steadying the burden as the lift trundled over to the waiting truck. Cissy, Blue Bell's first charge and her favorite, walked close to the horse's head. The girl talked to Blue Bell constantly and the horse seemed to pay attention, for she lay submissively and quietly as she was carried over to her makeshift ambulance. By means of buttons, switches and levers, Angelo raised Blue Bell's mattress to the level of the back of the truck. He moved the fork-lift forward a few feet, so that the horse was over the floor of the truck, and carefully, very carefully, the men slowly slid the plywood off the fork and onto the truck.

"So far, so good," Mr. Bemis muttered as he wiped his forehead with his hand. He was sweating and flushed with his efforts and his constant fear that the horse might become panicky, fall off the lift and break a leg. He kept glancing around among the sea of faces every so often to make sure I was on hand.

The funeral procession began.

The fork-lift led the way. Mr. Bemis drove the truck and young Bert was seated next to him in the driver's cab. Cissy, Benjie and Roy rode in the truck bed along with the horse. The youngsters' quiet presence comforted the beast. Mr. Bemis drove slowly and took the bumps on the road carefully.

I drove my car next in line; Mrs. Bemis followed me in the family car and Grandma and Grandpa Bemis came next. Our little procession wound its way down the road. All the neighbors were out in their front yards or on their porches, and they waved goodbye as we passed. One or two couples jumped into their car and took their place behind the senior Bemises. I never saw anything like it.

A mile or so up the road, a large back-hoe joined the funeral line, and three miles later we passed the mandrake groves once again and reached the farm. Old Mr. Purdy, hat in hand, and all the children I had seen that first time I had attended Blue Bell, were on hand. They were all a year older but the scene was much as it was before.

The Bemis children jumped down from the truck and the menfolk took their positions by the rear gate of the vehicle, which they lowered to receive the fork-lift.

The back-hoe went on its way to a field full of daisies close by. It began to dig a hole.

Angelo carefully carried Blue Bell and deposited her on her pallet just inside the barn door. There was no need to carry her back into the barn to her old stall. Near the door, where it was more open, she could smell the sweet air and feel the early-morning sun. Anxious faces and willing hands gently settled the mattress and its burden on the old barn floor.

Blue Bell knew she was home. She raised her head, sniffed the wisteria and lilac-scented air, whinnied appreciatively, and with another little nicker, laid her great head on a pillow of sweet hay. It made the Bemises' magnificent effort all that much more worthwhile, for it was a whinny of recognition, appreciation and contentment.

My services, fortunately, had not been needed, so I patted Blue Bell, said goodbye to her and then said my goodbyes to the Bemis family.

Mr. Bemis wanted to pay me for my time, but I wouldn't hear of it. I was glad to have been on hand just in case, but I hadn't done anything. He tried to hand me a twenty-dollar bill, but I gently pushed his hand back and he dropped the money accidentally. The bill fluttered to the ground and he stooped to retrieve it, ripping up a clover blossom that got pinched in the fold of the bill.

"No, Mr. Bemis—please, no. Not this time."

A phone call the next morning at ten brought the sad news that Blue Bell had just died.

I had never been to a funeral for a horse before; it was very moving. The fork-lift once again carried Blue Bell, this time to the grave site, a huge hole which the back-hoe had dug the day before. It must have been a good ten feet deep and ten feet square. Another friend with heavy equipment appeared now—this one had a hoist. They secured chains around either end of the plywood and carefully lifted the animal and its bed into the air. Four men steadied the burden to keep it from swaying. These were Blue Bell's pallbearers, I thought, and suddenly Honilee appeared in my mind's eye. . . . Honilee hadn't received half the love.

There was a gentle breeze, and all the leaves and flowers gave sad little nods. Everything was quiet; all that could be heard was the clinking of chains. The small crane swung Blue Bell around, positioned her over the hole and slowly lowered the plywood, the mattress and Blue Bell down into the grave. I blinked and sniffed and tasted salt, felt the grass and smelled the flowers, saw the trees and heard the people, and as I studied Blue Bell I knew we would all be grass again and we are all one in that common chain—that bond that links all living things.

After the grave was covered over, Cissy, Benjie, Roy and Bert planted a young tree on top of the mound.

"An apple tree—a young apple tree for Blue Bell," Mrs. Bemis whispered to me, tears streaming down her cheeks. "I'll never forget how Blue Bell loved to snooze under her favorite apple tree." She took a deep breath and wiped her wet cheeks.

The only thing missing was organ music, and I'm glad they hadn't provided any, for I'm sure I would have been overcome. Even so, I had all I could do to control myself when the kids sang "Rock of Ages."

After the funeral, Mrs. Bemis served coffee and homemade breads and cakes. We were seated around a large oval kitchen table, and the construction workers, some dipping their bread into their coffee before taking a bite, were discussing how smoothly everything had gone. Mrs. Bemis sat between Dr. Ferris and me. Dr. Ferris was old enough to be my grandfather, but he was still practicing, and was still hale and hearty. I wondered if that's what having a large-animal practice did for a person, and perhaps my leaving it would prove to be a mistake. Anyway, I hoped I would look as good as he did when I reached his age. He must have retained a sentimentality about his profession over all his years, for I had noticed that his eyes were not completely dry when they were lowering Blue Bell away. Somehow this made me admire the tough old man more and it comforted me to know that I was not the only soft-hearted vet around.

Dr. Ferris was nodding and smiling recognition as Mrs. Bemis showed him a worn photograph in a small album. The picture was of a horse with a tiny tow-headed little girl on top.

"I remember." He nodded again. "That's Cissy. She must have been two or so, from the looks of her." Dr. Ferris glanced at the other pictures.

"Look, Dr. Logue," said Mrs. Bemis, turning toward me. "This is how Blue Bell used to look in her prime."

I saw all kinds of pictures. In one photo, Blue Bell had three children on her back. In another, she was looking down at a creature between her front feet; it was a small child. The album was a complete record of Blue Bell, all the Bemis children and how they grew.

"My, how Blue Bell loved little children," Mrs. Bemis stated, pouring Dr. Ferris a second cup of coffee. "Babies could play beneath her and crawl between her legs and never once was she so clumsy she'd harm them with her hoofs. She would look down at them and she would shift her hoof just so." The woman sighed sadly. "There will never be another Blue Bell."

And there never would.

I drove home more slowly than usual. Perhaps "reluctantly" would be a better way to phrase it.

I studied every verdant hill, every flowering field, every graceful turn in the road. I was at odds with myself. I was seeing these things for the last time; I was seeing them for the first time. Though glad that I was still in Kingston for Blue Bell's last call, I was sorry I had been there. Creatures like Blue Bell made it very difficult for me to leave my large-animal practice; people like the Bemises made it harder still. All I could remember at the moment were all the happy times—the Hansens and their Brown Swiss herd, the Boldingers and their goats, Nate Adams and his sheep, and the Wassenmuellers and my wedding ring, which I lost inside their cow while delivering a calf. These were the folks who filled my mind, and I could hardly remember now the Stemmlers and the Kidneys.

I was driving along Esopus Creek. It meandered and wound along its way until it reached the city limits, where we parted company as it continued under a narrow bridge and I made a left turn and drove up the hill. I passed the abandoned red-brick church which was standing alone and sadly forgotten with its broken stained-glass windows. There was a sudden kindled flare as a truant ray of sunshine flickered through the splintered remains of a piece of red glass, and then it was gone.

I made a right turn onto Foxhall Avenue, another onto Albany, and I was home.

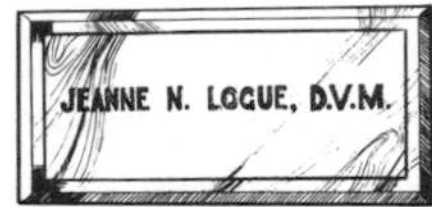

21

The closing took place as scheduled on a Wednesday afternoon, and when we returned home Joe called, "Well, it's all over, kids! We'll finish what packing we plan to do ourselves and the movers come tomorrow to finish the main part of the job. The next day we move. Friday night we'll be in our new house!"

I had never seen Joe so happy and ebullient! All the past week after he returned from work, he'd turned on the record player and played "This Old House." He played it over and over and he danced to it, around and around, arms raised over his head, fingers snapping smartly in rhythm to the music. Over and over he'd play the damn thing till I was near crazed. For some maddening reason, the happier Joe acted, the more miserable I became.

Thursday evening was to be the last one in my office. I had worked the past week with the new owner and had introduced him to a number of my large-animal clients and to the owners of the smaller pets who had come to the office. John, divorced from Debbie by now, and Agnes Brown, who replaced Debbie, planned to stay on, but Mame was going to retire, for the new doctor already had a tried and true tireless assistant of his own—his wife.

There was an affectionate goodbye when Mame left late

Thursday afternoon. Raymond, trailed by Marilyn, went out back toward the boarding kennel to take a last look at the young sycamore tree he had planted and given to me for a birthday present one year. He wished he could dig it up and take it with him. He sadly pushed the old black inner-tube swing, which was beginning to crack and deteriorate with age, and as he watched it sway idly, he remembered many things.

Even old Star was sad. She moped through the house like a lost soul. She could not settle down, but paced from room to room with a worried air, for the animal sensed that a change was about to take place.

There was a funerary attitude around the dinner table that evening and everyone ate Mame's last meal, a casserole so as not to dirty a lot of pots and pans, in glum silence. Joe alone was in good spirits and I guess he was a little disappointed in the attitude of the rest of the family. He was happy and he wanted to share it with somebody.

"Tomorrow's moving day!" He beamed.

"Just think," I said, feeling I ought to try to work up a little enthusiasm. "This Saturday morning I am going to bake an apple pie for everybody!"

"Really? In the *morning,* Mom?" asked Marilyn. "Well! I just can't picture you in the kitchen in the morning instead of being on a farm call or in the operating room or treating animals in the office!"

"Why not?" I laughed. "We'll have plenty of time for doing things together. This night marks the end of two-o'clock-in-the-morning pie-baking episodes for your mother."

"Why don't you learn to make apple strudel?" asked Ray.

"Why don't you write a book?" asked Joe.

I put my knife down and looked at him, seated across the table from me.

"That sounds like a very good idea," I said quietly.

"But wait a minute! What about all the animals?" wailed

Marilyn, as if suddenly realizing all that was being left behind.

"We're leaving all the animals here in the hospital, Maryl," Joe tried to explain. "Don't you understand? We're not going to have any more hospital. No more phones ringing—no more animals."

"You mean," Marilyn asked him, "that Mother isn't going to be a doctor at all anymore? You mean that Mother is going to be just a mother?"

"Jees, Marilyn, what do you mean?" Raymond placed his glass of milk down carefully and slowly, as if to emphasize his words. "What do you mean—*just* a mother?"

The profound meaning behind my son's words was as a balm to a wound. He recruited my spirits and suddenly I felt as tall as a mountain and very, very proud. The move didn't seem so bad at all to me anymore.

In the office that last evening, Mrs. Wilson was beside herself with grief. Little Mimi, who once had a vaginal polyp, was growing old. Her muzzle had turned gray and she had lost most of her teeth. Mimi had developed senile cataracts, which were inoperable, but the little dog got around the house well in spite of being blind, because Mrs. Wilson never moved the furniture and Mimi was so familiar with the traffic pattern of the house that she never bumped into anything.

"What will Mimi do when her time comes?" Mrs. Wilson lamented.

I had the deepest sympathy for the woman, because within her own scheme of priorities and values, Mrs. Wilson was as genuinely concerned about the welfare of this one small creature as some people would be about a small child.

Honilee came to my mind again and with her also the thought: If only she could have received some small portion of the love Mrs. Wilson has lavished on Mimi . . .

Mrs. Wilson continued, "Oh, Doctor, whatever will we do

without you? How shall we manage? If Mimi ever gets so that she can't hold her water, or is in pain, I'll have to have her put to sleep, for I couldn't stand to see her suffer. I can't bear to think of anyone but you doing that last final act. Mimi knows and loves you. She's afraid of strangers. You have such a way with animals." And she started weeping all over again.

All over the world, if a dog is coddled and pampered, it is usually the Pekingese or the toy poodle. There is something about these small, more exotic breeds that seems to have an affinity to a certain type of human personality. That was the style twenty years ago, and nowadays we can add to that list the Lhasa apso, the pug and the papillon.

I tried my best to comfort the poor woman, remembering that arthritic little Mimi was the only living being she had. "Please try not to feel so bad, Mrs. Wilson. That final act you dread may never have to be done, but if the time arrives and you believe it is necessary, I know you will find the new doctor very gentle and very understanding. I'm sure, in time, Mimi will get to trust and like him too." I couldn't think of anything more to say, but decided to end our morbid discussion with a lighter thought. I smiled at her and squeezed her hand. "You know, Mrs. Wilson, veterinarians love animals too. Now, what seems to be the problem with Mimi tonight?"

Carefully Mrs. Wilson stood Mimi on the table for me to see. The dog had an ingrown toenail which had grown so long that it had curled around back on itself and punctured the pad, causing it to swell and exude pus. It was apparently quite painful and Mimi had started limping on it that afternoon. I asked Mrs. Wilson to hold Mimi in her arms so that I could remove the ingrown length of nail. I cleaned out the puncture wound and told her that the pad would heal quickly now that the nail was removed. She asked for that darling little girl who used to spay her dolls, and I told her that Marilyn was fine and that she was quite a grown-up girl now, in third grade.

Mrs. Wilson had dried her tears and seemed to be feeling a bit more cheerful. She said she wondered at how time flies and told me how shocked she was when Marilyn told her that the doll wasn't sick at all and that she was just going to spay it. We both laughed, each of us recalling the incident clearly, as if it had happened only yesterday. . . .

The office was empty.

I thought of what I had to do next and I experienced a cowardly moment. Sinking wearily into my desk chair, I gazed up at the wall and tried to gather courage to march down the driveway and take down my shingle. My eyes fell upon license number 1582 affixed to the wall. "Be it known," the words were printed, "that Jeanne Neubecker Logue, having given satisfactory evidence of fitness . . . was examined and found duly qualified to receive this license to practice Veterinary Medicine and Surgery. . . ."

I turned out the lights and then I stifled a sob and converted it to a sigh as I flipped the switch for the light that illuminated my shingle out front. I tiptoed down the driveway in the darkness, hoping desperately that no one would turn into the driveway and catch me in the act. I worked almost furtively in the dark, as if I were committing an evil deed. At last I got the sign unhooked, and with trembling hands, took my shingle down.

I'll never forget how surprisingly heavy the sign seemed to me as I carried it back toward my office, and that night I dreamed a most morbid dream. I dreamed that I was lost and wandering around aimlessly, wondering where to hide the dead child that I suddenly found I was carrying in my arms.

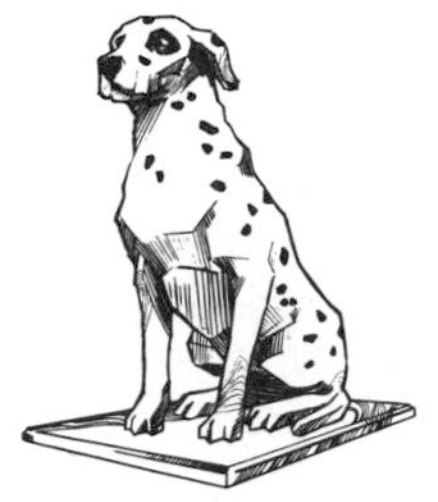

22

Our property was not all that had been sold. The land almost opposite ours, all wooded with tall and aged trees, was going to be used as the site of a shopping center. Any day the bulldozers would come, and since the practice had been sold, I'd been hoping we'd be packed and gone before they started clearing the land. I didn't want to see those trees come down.

The buzz saws and bulldozers arrived just as the movers were finishing with the loading of our furniture, and the clickety-click of Star's nails on the bare floors made such a lonesome sound.

Finally the movers rolled out of the driveway, and as the children, the dog and I followed in our car, the first tree was felled. I heard a fearful cracking like the breaking of some mammoth bone. I looked back only once. My favorite elm tree had been the first to go and its death left two gaping holes of emptiness—one along the skyline and the other in my heart.

Now my days were filled with gentler pursuits. I remember one day when Marilyn, for the first time in her life, saw me behind an ironing board. "Oh, Mother!" There was a new respect and an admiration in her voice. "I didn't know that you knew how to *iron ruffled curtains!*" And then there was Raymond returning from school, bursting into the kitchen like a gust of March wind. *Bang!* The screen door.

"Ma?" he shouted.

"I'm right here, Raymond. You don't have to shout. What is it you want?"

"Oh. Hi, Ma. I don't want anything. I just like to call 'Ma' when I come in and hear you answer. It's so nice to have you here when I come home."

Joe very magnanimously helped me with my plans for a third child, and it seemed no time at all before we were on our way to the hospital, with Joe tense and worried and driving very fast. I was about to tell him to relax, when, unable to contain himself any longer, he blurted out, "Jesus H. Christ! Don't you dare make a mess of this car!"

The next thing I knew, the bright delivery room lights were over my head. There were beaming faces all about, then a resounding smack, a lusty wail and a warm wiggling weight laid on my abdomen as the doctor clamped and tied the unbilical cord.

"It's a boy, Mrs. Logue. A fine baby boy!" said the nurse, who was wreathed in smiles. I vaguely heard the doctor's voice—something about checking me to be sure. He had heard a double heartbeat, and was mumbling to the nurse about the possibility of twins.

"You mean you're not sure? A bouncer like she just had and you aren't sure?" asked the nurse. Her white cap bobbed like a little dove as she shook her head and looked archly at the doctor.

"Hmm. Evidently it was just an echo beat I heard."

"Some doctor you are," the nurse continued to tease. "Some diagnostician. Why, I wouldn't even take my dog to you!"

"You know, I wouldn't either," my doctor agreed with her, and winking at me, he tweaked my big toe and added, "I'd take my dog to a veterinarian!"

It was springtime once again. A wrack of high clouds in a wind-driven mass raced across the sky, hid the sun for a moment and then rushed onward as if suddenly caught in a strong riptide of current. I was returning from a trip to Kingston. One of Ralph Dorsey's horses was lame and as an old friend I went to see what I could do to help. Actually, I was surprised at the number of clients who "followed" me from Kingston. While I did not have a full-time practice anymore, I still was not completely out of it. There were frequent phone calls either for advice or to make an appointment to drive down to Poughkeepsie to see me and have me examine their animals and treat those I could, considering my present medical setup.

Raymond was just returning from crew as I pulled into the driveway.

"First day in the shell out on the river," he called to me. "This year Arlington is going to have the winning crew! School's fun all of a sudden, Ma. Somehow I don't mind studying anymore. Even Shakespeare seems to make sense nowadays. I suppose that means I'm growing up."

We entered the kitchen together and our nostrils were greeted with the delicious aroma of a freshly baked apple pie.

"I wanted to surprise you!" Marilyn said gaily. She was outlined against the kitchen window, her cheeks flushed from the heat of the kitchen and her dark hair shining with tinges of red from the last rays of the setting sun. I often wondered how I could have hatched anything so completely feminine as Marilyn. I had always been such a tomboy myself and as I look back on my childhood I wonder how my mother could have stood me at times.

I kissed her. "You make the best pies, Maryl. Where's Paul?"

"Down in the woods with Star, exploring."

I had just finished preparing dinner when a four-year-old figure clad in brown trousers and boots flashed by the window and opened the kitchen door. Nature boy was back and I wondered where his black boots and blue trousers had gone. I rolled my eyes heavenward and put a hand on my forehead as I realized Paul still wore his original clothes and that they had turned brown because of a thick coating of mud. I could hear it squush inside his boots as he stepped into the kitchen, and I watched in silent despair as it dripped slowly, like sewer sludge, down his pants and onto the clean floor. Now I knew how I must have looked the night I was christened by Curly Hurley's cow while I was giving it a rectal exam.

Paul stopped on a dime. One hand went up, and with palm opened and fingers together, he patted the air as if giving a benediction.

"Peace be with you," the gesture implied. "Be calm!" it implored. "Hold your tongue." Such an eloquent motion; I knew exactly what it meant, for in his short span of time, Paul had perfected his own silent form of communication. I waited patiently; I knew what his next words would be.

"Hear me out!" The hand patted the air again, and he tilted his head back slightly and closed his eyes as he continued his supplication.

"Hear me out!" I swore the boy was going to grow up and become a preacher. I could hear and see him now in his pulpit. I don't know why I suddenly loved him so much at that moment, but I did.

I heard Paul out. One hand had remained in his pocket all during his pantomime, but he withdrew it now, carefully extracting a new find.

"I got a little creature here, Ma," and I immediately changed my mind about the preacher bit and decided he was going to become a psychologist instead, the way he intuitively knew how to get to a body. Naturally, I melted and was immediately involved. We all were, and with mud and mess forgotten, all four of us bent in rapt attention over Paul's newly found creature. What was it this time?

Paul slowly opened his palm and there it was—hard and round and a dull green. It was a turtle, a baby snapping turtle.

In spite of its smallness, it already had a ferocious look as it glowered out at us from the protection of its shell. The piercing eyes were an evil yellow, hostile and unblinking. The turtle slowly extended his relatively large head and long serpentlike tail, and then hissed and retreated again as Paul startled him by a sudden movement of his hand.

Ray ferreted out a large turtle dish from the miscellaneous supply of pet cages and tanks stored in the basement, and soon the turtle was in his new home, which Ray landscaped with a little cave made of small rocks, some twigs and a supply of mud and water. I offered the turtle a small chunk of raw meat. He remained motionless, eying my hand with a measured malevolence as we waited to see what he would do.

Suddenly, *flash! Snap!* A sharp beaklike mouth attached to a very long neck darted at me and tore the meat from my fingers. I never dreamed that the little fellow could move so fast or that he could reach so far. We continued to observe the turtle as he ripped and tore at the meat, tugging with his head and neck as his sharp claws shredded the chunk into bite-size gulpable pieces. There was not one gentle aspect about its entire tiny being. The carnivorous reptile; it was all still there. One hundred fifty million years of living lurked within that one tiny shell.

"I'll let him go free again after a week or so," Paul said as he started up the stairs to change his clothes and wash for dinner.

Ray had his nose in an encyclopedia.

"O.K., everybody. I've found the turtle's name," and he pasted a label on the turtle tank which read: IN RESIDENCE—CHELYDRA SERPENTINA.

During dinner that night Ray and Marilyn started reminiscing about the Kingston days and all the animals, and Paul felt he had missed something. For Paul the animal business was very new and he always looked forward to a sick animal's coming to the house.

"Can't I ride with you the next time you go on a call, Ma? Maryl says she used to." And so I promised him that he could go with me the very next call I made.

He did not have long to wait, for one day soon after I made this promise, the phone rang, and while the tearful voice I heard was somehow familiar, it was so distorted by grief that I could not identify it.

There were a series of sobs and finally a familiar, "Dr. Logue?"

"Yes, speaking."

"Oh, Doctor, I just can't bear it. I cannot bear to see her suffer." There were more sobs. "This is Mrs. Wilson, Doctor. It's my little Mimi—" And now she cried uncontrollably. She finally quieted down enough for me to learn that Mimi's time had come.

"She's all swollen, Dr. Logue. Mimi has dropsy. The heart pills and diuretic she's taking just don't seem to do any good anymore. She can hardly get around and she has a terrible time breathing—she's just constantly fighting for air. I know she is suffering and I can't bear it." She sobbed again, but soon got on with it. "It's time for Mimi to be put to sleep. Mimi has never quite taken to the new doctor, so couldn't you please, wouldn't you please, please come and take care of her here at home? Oh, please, Dr. Logue?" she begged. "Just this one last time."

"Of course, Mrs. Wilson," I said gently. "Of course I'll come."

It was one of those beautiful old stone houses out in Hurley which dated back to the 1700s. Remnants of an old-fashioned garden evoked memories of a bygone age. Flower-bordered paths, graceful and inviting, wound their way leisurely around one bend and then onto another, and each successive curve displayed azaleas, tulips and daffodils blooming in profusion.

In the distance could be seen dried spires of hollyhocks, the sentinels of summer past.

I saw a huge stone carriage block by the side of the driveway, under the portico. A heavy iron ring still dangled from one end, the kind they used to tether horses. I envisioned a horse and carriage pulling up, a door opening and a lady in a hoop skirt stepping carefully out and onto the stone.

The immense living room was dominated by a wide curving staircase made of golden oak. It seemed to flow from the floor above down into the center of the room. There were also two fine old clocks, both standing with great self-esteem, tall and erect like two proud aristocrats. Their backs were held stiffly against opposite walls so that they were facing each other. The larger of the two was a ponderous grandfather clock with all manner of gears inside him and with little windows in his face so that in addition to the time, he accounted for the date and the phases of the moon. He had a rather masculine, authoritative sound and went *toc, toc.* The grandmother clock standing opposite was slim and dainty in comparison. She had blue forget-me-nots and tiny pink rosebuds in smiling garlands around her face, and the tips of her elegant hands were manicured with gold leaf. She was mistress of the gentler moments, ticking off the minutes and the hours with a refined *tic, tic.*

Over the mantle, surrounded by an ornate golden openwork frame was an oval picture, a wedding portrait of Mr. and Mrs. Wilson. I looked at the serious-faced young man and the smiling smooth-browed bride. I could hardly recognize the young lady as the same woman who was sitting on the velvet sofa now, puffy-eyed, swollen-lipped and blotchy-faced from crying.

The two clocks were keeping the vigil together—*toc, toc* and *tic, tic.* Both pairs of hands pointed as one now, for it was three-fifteen.

Mimi's time had come.

I went over to the little dog lying on Mrs. Wilson's comfortable lap. Mimi had her chin elevated and extended, and was resting it on the low arm of the sofa. This seemed to make her chore of breathing a bit easier.

Wheeze in, huff out—wheeze and huff. Her breathing sounds filled the room.

"Mimi?" I called her and then stroked her shining head. "Mimi? Remember me?"

Rheumy eyes turned toward me. I spoke her name again. Mimi perked up her ears and wagged her tail!

"My word! I believe Mimi remembers me, Mrs. Wilson."

"Well, you know Mimi always was a smart little dog, and she always loved you, Doctor."

There was no question about it. After all the time that had passed, the little dog still remembered me! The tail wag was no mere polite gesture, it was an act of positive recognition; Mimi licked my hand with her warm little cyanotic tongue.

"Here, let me take her, Mrs. Wilson."

"I can't bear to watch. I just can't bear it," and she added distractedly, "But then—oh, dear, I really shouldn't leave Mimi at this last moment, should I?" Mrs. Wilson's face went blank and her voice took on an odd, expressionless sound. "Tell me what to do. I don't know what to do."

"Why don't you and Paul go out in the garden a moment? If Mimi seems upset by your being gone, I'll call you. If she seems content, I'll just put her to sleep." And then to Paul, "Take Mrs. Wilson down some of those garden paths, Paul. See what flowers are in bloom."

He took the poor woman by the hand and led her out of doors into the spring sunshine. They paused a moment in the sun and I could hear some of Paul's conversation.

"We have petunias in our yard, Mrs. Wilson, and you know what my job was when they were first planted? My job was to put mothballs around them to keep the rabbits away. Small plants got two mothballs and bigger ones got three."

"Mothballs?"

"Yes, Mrs. Wilson. And you know what? Sometimes it was a very hard job. You know why?"

"No, I don't, dear. Why was it hard sometimes?"

"Well," Paul explained patiently, "sometimes when I got to an in-between-sized plant, I couldn't decide if it was a two- or three-baller!"

I smiled at his words, vividly recalling his small figure out in our garden, clad in red overalls and clutching his bag of mothballs, bogged down in his progress by decisions, decisions.

Mimi was curled in her special little bed by the fireplace. It was all over for her now and the room was blessedly quiet as I put my hypodermic away. I went to call Paul and Mrs. Wilson.

"But when are you going to—you know—do it, Dr. Logue?"

"It's all over, Mrs. Wilson. Mimi is gone."

"She is?" Mrs. Wilson looked bewildered. "But she looks just as if she is sleeping."

"She is, in a way." I smiled sympathetically and closed my bag.

"Yes, yes. I realize that now. The room seems so quiet all of a sudden. It's almost a relief." She was still holding one of Paul's hands in both her own, squeezing it gently now and then. She seemed to hate to let it go.

"What shall I do? Whatever shall I do? I'll be all alone in this house tonight, all alone."

"But you still have your handyman, Perce, and his wife, Ella, with you, don't you?" I asked.

"Yes, but—" And then she sighed and asked if we'd stay for tea.

She looked over her teacup a bit wistfully at Paul, who was joining us with a glass of milk and a cookie.

"Oh, how I wish I had had a nice little boy like you—and

a little girl like your sister, Marilyn, who always spayed her dolls." She shook her head sadly. "That was a joy Mr. Wilson and I were never privileged to have . . . and I am so sorry. It's too bad, you know, because I believe we would have made good parents."

"Oh, I think so too, Mrs. Wilson," Paul agreed. He pointed a small thumb at his chest and said, "I *know* you would!"

"I'm sure you would too, Mrs. Wilson." I patted her hand, despairing of how to comfort her. "You have so much love and wisdom to give. I know of one little girl who could have used some of your love." I was thinking of Honilee.

"I want your children to have something to remember me by." Seeming to brighten slightly, she left the room and returned shortly carrying a box. There was an ancient silk fan for Marilyn. It was embroidered with roses which were still unfaded in spite of all the years and very beautiful. The stays were made of ivory.

"I used it at a cotillion—my first grand ball! We kept changing partners, but Mr. Wilson always sought me out."

For Paul there was a small toy fire engine. It was carved out of wood and all moving parts worked smoothly. A small wood carving of a fire dog, a black-and-white Dalmatian, was for Paul too.

To Raymond Mrs. Wilson gave a handsome bone letter opener with intricate engravings on it.

"That's walrus bone," she explained. "It is a fine example of the art of scrimshaw. It used to be my husband's."

"But, Mrs. Wilson, surely you don't want to part with such sentimental possessions. I—"

"That is exactly why I want to part with them. I want to give something of great value to me. It will comfort me some way, knowing your children have them. It makes me feel as though I'll be in closer touch somehow. . . ."

On the way home, Paul sat next to me on the front seat, pensively turning one of the wooden wheels of his fire engine. I had tried to persuade him to stay home, explaining the nature of the visit to Mrs. Wilson and the fact that it would be a sad one, but he had wanted to come along anyway. After all, I had promised.

"Don't feel so bad about Mimi, Paul. The little dog had a very happy life—happier than some people do. She was sick and suffering and the thing you must remember is that she is not suffering anymore."

"Oh, I'm not so unhappy about the dog, Mother, but I feel so sad for Mrs. Wilson. She's all alone now. All she has are those two old clocks that keep talking to each other."

"You know, you're right, Paul. Those two clocks did seem to be talking across the room to each other. Imagine! They have probably been carrying on a conversation for over one hundred years."

"I wonder if they ever had an argument?" And our imaginations were carried away. We decided that when the clocks argued, that's what caused them to run fast. If one or the other sulked, the clock would run slow.

"Well, anyway, Mother, I'm going to find Mrs. Wilson a new pet—a new pet to keep her company."

His face took on a "bright idea" look; I knew he had discovered something.

"You know what, Mother? I just figured something. Mrs. Wilson just needs something to love, that's all. *Everybody* needs something to love."

"Would you like to stop in at a farm where I used to treat cattle?" I asked, hoping to end the day on a happier note. We were on Route 9W in Esopus, nearing Rosenthal Lane. I used to make many calls to this farm and it would be nice to stop in and say a quick hello.

Everything looked so different from my memory of it. A line of motels had been built on the farm and I recalled the motel sign on the main road. REST IN QUIET COMFORT, it read, with an arrow pointing down Rosenthal Lane. I was disappointed not to find the owner home, so I contented myself by showing Paul the barns and the cattle. It was just about milking time and a hired man was getting the milking machines ready. He must have been behind schedule, for the cows, with full udders, were bawling and lowing, voicing their growing discomfort.

All I could see was the man's broad, blue-jeaned backside as he bent over his work. He was noisily rinsing out milking cups as we entered, and he turned as he heard us. His face became enlivened with recognition.

"I remember you!" He slapped his thigh. "Sure, I remember you—you're the lady vet who used to come here all the time." And suddenly it was like old times and we were discussing mastitis, milk fever, ketosis, and I was smelling familiar smells. I suppressed a wave of nostalgia and longing and refused to give way to such a peculiar form of homesickness. I was glad to find this familiar face, for there is nothing that is more of a letdown than to return to a place after a number of years, a place where you used to belong, and find it all changed about, with new people who treat you as a trespasser and a stranger.

"Little boy." The hired man grinned a chin-stubbled smile at Paul. "Didja ever have a drink of milk right from the cow?"

"No, only from milk bottles the milkman leaves. It's good fresh milk." Paul boasted as if he were the owner of the dairy.

"Would you like some right from the cow, sonny?"

"Well—" Paul stammered as he eyed the cow and the hired man attaching the milking cups to the teats. "Well—are you sure that's fresh milk?"

"Fresh milk?" The stubby face was creased into smiles. "How can you get milk any fresher, son? See? It's straight from the cow," and he reached for the udder next in the milking line and shot a white stream across the floor.

"But maybe that cow wasn't milked yesterday and she's got day-old milk."

Paul was fascinated by the large animals and I was glad I had taken the time to stop by. It ended his day happily and besides, the child learned something new, least of which was the fact that the milk was fresh and that it was delivered warm.

On the trip home, Paul was full of talk.

"Mother, do cows really have four stomachs?"

"No, they really have just one with four separate compartments, although each compartment is always referred to as a stomach. Each stomach has a different function and does its own job. The first three stomachs are named the rumen, the reticulum and the omasum. They have no gastric glands, but the fourth one, the abomasum or true stomach, does."

We arrived home a bit later than I had expected and I immediately began to prepare dinner. Paul asked me to tell him once again about the farmer and the lightning bolt, and all the while I told him the story, my hands, which had cured the sick and healed the wounded, kept skillfully peeling potatoes. I told him how lightning once struck a farmer's barn and how the electricity was conducted through the metal stanchions and traveled the entire length of the barn, electrocuting every cow in every stanchion, one after the other right down the line, bowling them over like a row of toppling dominoes.

Joe brought an unexpected guest home for dinner and Paul went off, looking for Marilyn, sorry to have the story hour interrupted. He was eager now to tell her about poor Mrs. Wilson and little Mimi, and about the presents Mrs. Wilson had given them.

During dinner the phone rang and I excused myself to answer. When I returned to the table, I couldn't wait for dinner to be over, for the guest to leave and for the children to be in bed. I had just received an exciting phone call and I wanted to discuss it with Joe.

"Well, what do you think?" I asked. We had just settled down in bed and I rested my head on Joe's shoulder so we could talk.

"This is something you are going to have to decide for yourself," Joe answered. "If you want to, go ahead and accept this doctor's offer and join him. The only thing I don't want to happen is to have us go back to a schedule as busy and as hectic as we used to have in Kingston. That's the only stipulation I'm going to make. I'm dumping the whole decision in your lap!" He kissed me and added, "It's your nickel!"

"I told him I'd think about it, discuss it with you and then let him know."

"Is that what you told him? You'd let him know?" Joe laughed in the darkness. He dislodged me as he propped himself up on his elbow and continued. "I'll tell you, Jeanne. I'll tell you exactly what you are going to do. You are going to agonize over all the pros and cons, the why you shoulds and the why you shouldn'ts, and after you go through your ritualistic dance, you are going to accept his offer."

Epilogue

Joe was right. I did agonize for about a week before I returned that telephone call and became Dr. Logue once more.

While working for another veterinarian was not the same as conducting my own practice, it was, all in all, a happy solution. My days could not have been busier, for whether conducting my own practice or someone else's, after all, there is just so much surgery one can do in one day. I did miss the large-animal work and I will admit that there were times when I contemplated starting up a new practice of my own again and not confining myself to just small-animal medicine. But such daydreams were always put aside and I pragmatically said no to myself. It was an era of fast economic growth and Joe and I always lived under the shadow of IBM's transferring us to either Boulder, Colorado, or San Jose, California, or wherever, for the corporation was expanding rapidly and there was much moving about of personnel. I never planted an autumn tulip, daffodil or hyacinth bulb but what I wondered if I would be there the following spring to see it bloom. If Joe was transferred to the West Coast it would be a relatively simple matter as a salaried veterinarian to tender a resignation, rather than, having got involved in a practice of my own, go through the process of selling a specialized piece of real estate. Besides, I had been through all that once before and wished no part of it again, for whatever reason. Under these circumstances, I wouldn't consider a practice even on a partnership basis. But I was very happy just to be able to practice veterinary medicine, and as I look back on all the changes that have taken place in the field during the past thirty years, I am exceedingly proud to have been part of the growth of the profession. I often compare the early days of practicing to the early days of flying, when there were the barnstormers, the pilots who used to fly by the seat of their pants, so to speak. They depended more on their intuitive abilities and a compass than on control towers, computers and a lot of fancy instruments, as nowadays. Veterinarians, too, used to practice more by the seat of their pants. We depended on our *senses* more than we do now. We diagnosed more by *seeing, hearing* and *smelling* the symptoms; we just had to *know,* that's all, and for all the crude practices that used to be, we still got some pretty good results. Before my time, veterinarians used even their sense of *taste* as a diagnostic aid: the real old-timers confirmed diabetes mellitis by dipping a finger into a cow's urine specimen and tasting it. Now we have all manner of sophisticated laboratory aids and digital monitory devices, do EKGs on both large and small animals and catheterize their hearts. Thank heaven for the new anesthesia machines and their fine control of newer volatile gases, so that anesthetizing animals, humans included, is now a much safer procedure. We have artificial hip joints now, and a prosthesis for the knee is on its way. We have air-conditioned hospitals, some with a central oxygen source which can be tapped into individual cages as needed.

Veterinary medicine has come a long, long way, but that is not all that has changed over the years; our family has changed too.

It will not be too many more years before Joe will retire from IBM. He is still flying his own airplane and to my mind is the best pilot in the world. I would fly with him anywhere.

Raymond is married now to our lovely Antoinette and he has started his own corporation, Logue Avionics Ltd. He has invented and is marketing digital navigational instruments for aircraft.

Marilyn is married too, and is now Mrs. Dean Bartlett. Dr. Bartlett is an orthodontist and is practicing in Glens Falls, New York. They have two children, a girl and a boy. Marilyn has her teaching degree and is keeping a promise that she made to herself many years ago, when she was just a little girl.

I was tucking her in one night when we were still in Kingston and she confided that when she grew up and got married, she was going to arrange things so that her family would not be too busy. "I'm going to see to it that everybody takes time to enjoy one another," was the way she put it.

Paul has a little way to go yet. At present he is a student at Syracuse University and plans to become a dentist. It would not surprise me, however, if he changed his mind at the last minute and switched to one of the biological or natural sciences. He still brings the wild creatures home. With Paul, I feel as though I have completed some sort of life cycle, for I can honestly say to him what so often in the past clients said to me:

"You have such a way with animals."

Glossary

atrophy a reduction in size, a wasting due to lack of nutrition to any part.

auditory pertaining to the sense of hearing.

benign tumor a growth that is not recurrent, not malignant.

brucellosis infectious disease principally infecting cattle, swine, goats and man. Causes contagious abortion in cattle and undulant fever or malta fever in man.

carcinoma an epithelial cell new growth which may affect almost any organ or part of the body. Highly malignant with great tendency to metastasize.

carotid artery left and right, the principal vessels supplying blood to the neck and head.

connective tissue tissue concerned primarily with supporting bodily structures and holding parts together; for example, white and yellow C.T., cartilage and bone.

cornea the clear transparent portion coating the anterior surface of the eye.

cyanotic bluish, slatelike or dark purple discoloration of tissue due to a deficiency of oxygen and an excess of carbon dioxide.

distal farthest from the center or trunk; opposite of proximal.

diuretic an agent which increases the secretion of urine.
dystocia difficult labor, difficult delivery of a fetus.
electrolyte a solution which is a conductor of electricity. Acids, bases and salts are the common electrolytes.
emaciation state of being excessively lean.
embryotomy the dissection of a fetus to aid in its delivery.
emolient an agent that will soften and soothe.
enucleate to remove a part in its entirety.
euthanize ending a life easily, quietly and painlessly.
eviscerated having the internal ogans removed or protruding from the body cavity.
fascia a fibrous membrane supporting and separating muscle.
femoral pertaining to the thigh bone or femur.
fulminating occurring very rapidly.
gangrene death of tissue due to deficient or absent blood supply.
geld to castrate.
gonadotropin a substance having a stimulating effect on either the ovaries or testes.
hemangioma a benign tumor of the blood vessels.
hypercalcemia an excessive amount of calcium in the blood.
hypocalcemia abnormally low amount of calcium in the blood.
impaction condition of being tightly wedged, as feces in the bowel.
intercostal between the ribs.
intradermal within the structures of the skin.
intravenous within a vein.
jejunal arteries blood vessels supplying the second portion of the small intestine, that is, extending from the duodenum to the ileum.
lachrymal duct the duct which conveys tears.
lactation the function of secreting milk.

ligate to tie a blood vessel or other structure in order to constrict it.

lordosis abnormal convexity of the spine.

lumbar pertaining to the loins.

lumen space within an artery, vein, intestine or tube.

malignant tumor a growth that is cancerous, recurrent, not benign.

mesentery double fold of peritoneal membrane encircling the greater part of the small intestine and connecting the intestine to the posterior abdominal wall.

metastasize movement of bacteria or cells, especially cancer cells, from one part of the body to a new location.

milk fever paralysis, coma and death occurring after parturition caused by sudden drop in blood calcium level due to onset of profuse lactation.

necrosis death of tissue.

olfactory pertaining to the sense of smell.

optic pertaining to the sense of sight.

parturition act of giving birth to young.

peristaltic a progressive wavelike contraction of smooth muscle that occurs involuntarily in the alimentary canal.

prosthesis replacement of a missing part by an artificial substitute.

radial vein vessel removing blood from the forearm.

raphe a crease, ridge or seam noting the connection of the halves of a part.

resection partial excision of bone or other structures.

Ringer's lactate an aqueous solution of the electrolytes of sodium, potassium and calcium chloride and sodium lactate. It approximates the electrolyte concentration of the blood.

scours neonatal diarrhea.

septicemia blood poisoning due to invasion of the blood by bacteria or their toxins.

sternum the unpaired plate of bone forming the middle of the anterior wall of the chest.

subcutaneous beneath the skin.

torsion condition of being twisted.

tracheotomy operation of cutting into the trachea to overcome obstruction.

trochar a sharply pointed surgical instrument contained in a metal cannula.

tuberculin a sterile liquid containing the growth products extracted from the tubercle bacillus. Used in the diagnosis of tuberculosis infection.

umbilical ring a ring of connective tissue marking the scar of the former attachment of the umbilical cord to the fetus.

urachus fetal urinary canal.

vitreous body semisolid mass of a glasslike gel entirely filling the posterior chamber of the eye.

volvulus a twisting of the bowel on itself causing obstruction or strangulation.

Whartonian jelly a gelatinous intercellular substance consisting of primitive connective tissue of the umbilical cord.

withers the ridge between the shoulder blades. Those parts which resist the pull in drawing a load.